WEIGHT LOSS

INTRODUCTION

This book let you in on the Secrets of Why thin people are so thin? Is it hereditary or are they actually also struggling to maintain their weight? Weight loss is mostly about good habits,habits of eating mindfully,habit of taking the stairs rather than elevators sometime,habit of maintaining the habits for longterm like a marathon,rather than for short-term like a sprint.Aside from tips from thin people in chapter 1, Chapter 2 provide additional tips for dealing with weight loss,such as taking Multivitamins, dealing with depression,how to start fasting sometime.

Scientist discovered Why thin people dislike fat people-

The last chapter 3 deals with the scientific knowledge as well as controversy of weight loss.Yes science confusion about weight loss.Are thin people really healthy on the inside? Studies says thin people are a timebomb with lots of accumulated fat inside.How fat cells work,and why is it impossible to "burn" them off?Is there a molecular switch to turn off "Fat Switch?" Scientist discovered Why thin people dislike fat people. Why Thin Will Always Be In.9 Science-Backed Weight Loss Tips.**10 weight loss secrets from around the world.**

You will come out of this book having much more knowledge about the secrets of thin people, and realized that thin people does not have special abilities, but just good habits all along.And you will have additional knowledge about dealing with weight loss aside from thin people's secrets.Most of all ,the last chapter 3 about the science of weight loss will leave you with ideas,and theories and observation,and thinking about weight loss and thin people,etc,etc.

MORE IN DEPTH ON CHAPTER 1,2 AND 3. BUT YOU CAN JUST SKIP THIS

CHAPTER 1

23 Best-Ever Weight-Loss Secrets From Thin People

Some people can eat as much as they want and still stay slender. She eats an ice cream cone like there is no need to watch her weight, and she is right. And you know she always order meat, but she doesn't have superwoman genes either. So how come she can eat so much and yet remain as slim as before? "Diets don't work. They fail all the time," says Carla Heiser, a registered dietitian and certified specialist in nutritional and metabolic medicine in Chicago.And we discovered exactly the kind of secrets-of- secrets strategies you won't hear from nutritionist gurus and weight-loss doctors. Here are the rule-breaking secrets tricks that work for Thin people. Why not join the members of the Elite Group?

CHAPTER 2

Additional tip for weight loss such as how taking Multivitamins can helps in weight loss.How to cope with depression .How to reach out and stay connected. How to enjoy things.How to eat healthy.Get a healthy dose of sunlight.How to get professional help for depression.12 Popular weight loss pills and supplements.Fastings for beginners,learn to fast every now and then for a healthier you.How long can a person survive without food and water?

CHAPTER 3

Science research on weight loss and thin people, how fat cells work and why its impossible to "burn" them off.Are thin people really healthy on the inside?Is there a molecular switch to turn off obesity?why thin people dislike obese people?Weight loss secrets from around the world.How to loose 5 pound fast.Where to take vacation for weight loss.Science backed weight loss tips.

TABLE OF CONTENTS :

7) They Know hunger is not really an emergency :

8) Imagine Eating Before You Eat :

9) Thin People eat more fruits :

10) Thin people look after themselves first :

11) Thin People Exercise :

12) Thin People eat mindfully :

13) Thin People are creatures of habit :

14) Thin People have a Scale :

15)Thin People Don't waste time on diet foods :

16) No food is "bad." :

17)Thin People Step Away From the Screen :

18) An Apple a Day Melts the Pounds Away! :

19) Persistence is the key :

20) Thin people don't sit still :

21) Thin people live Outdoor :

22) Thin People take the stairs rather than the elevators to cut calories :

23) Add fun activities :
a) FRISBEE TOSS -
b) FETCH WITH FIDO -
c) VIRTUAL SPORTS -
d) Soccer Burns More Fat Than Jogging -

CHAPTER 2
ADDITIONAL WEIGHT LOSS TIPS

24) Take a Multivitamin :

25)Depression And Weight Gain:
a) Depression Leads to Weight Gain, Study Confirms -
b) Coping with Depression -
c) How to reach out for support to deal with your depression -
d) Tips for staying connected -
e) Do things that you like -
f) Look after your health -

26) Develop different kind of ways to deal with depression :
27) Exercise is something you can do right now to boost your mood :
28) Eat a healthy, depression-fighting diet :
29) Get a daily dose of sunlight :
30) Dealing with the winter blues :
31) Challenge negative thinking :
32) Put your thoughts on the witness stand :
33) When to get professional help for depression :
34) 12 Popular Weight Loss Pills and Supplements :

35) Intermittent Fasting And Weight Loss:
a) How Fasting At Irregular Intervals Can Help You Lose Weight-
b) How Irregular Fasting Change Your Hormones Positively-
a) Irregular Fasting Helps You Reduce Calories and Lose Weight-
b)Irregular Fasting May Help You To Hold On To Your Muscle-
c) Irregular Fasting Encourage Healthy Eating-
d)How to Succeed With an Irregular Fasting System-

36) Intermittent Fasting And Weight Loss:
a) Intermittent Fasting Helps You Reduce Calories and Lose Weight-
b) Intermittent Fasting May Help You To Hold On To Your Muscle -

c) Irregular Fasting Encourage Healthy Eating -
d)How to Succeed With an Irregular Fasting System-

37) How long can a person survive without food?
38) How long can humans survive without food or water?

CHAPTER 3

-

THE SCIENCE STUDY

39) Why its difficult to "burn off" belly fat,and how cell behaved :

40) Thin people may be fat on the inside, doctors warn :
a) Internal fat found in models-
b) Mistaken signals for fat storage-

41) Scientists discover why thin people dislike fat people:
42) Fat people are actually nicer than thin people, according to science:
43) Characteristics of metabolically unhealthy lean people:
44) Fat? Thin? Molecular switch may turn obesity on or off:
45) To Lose and Keep Off Weight, Turn Off Your Body's 'Fat Switch':
46) Is a Slim Physique Contagious? :
47) Obesity researchers study thin people for clues about hunger and metabolism :

CHAPTER 1

1) They Know It's Not a Sprint, Its A Marathon :

Maria Menounos says, "When I was forty pounds heavier and decided to lose the weight, I took a long-term, gradual approach. I didn't have the willpower to go on an extreme diet and drop all the foods I loved. And with work, paying the bills, my family and friends and my relationship, I certainly didn't have the time to exercise for two hours a day. It took a year or so, but I lost the forty pounds. Little did I know that slow and steady was not only the most realistic way to lose weight, but also the smartest. It's the main reason I never gained the weight back....The changes you make in your lifestyle can be slow and gradual and still get you where you want to go!"

2) They Don't Only Count the Calories :

Calories fuel our bodies, right? Actually, they don't. A calorie is simply a unit of measurment for heat; in the early 19th century, it was used to explain the theory of heat conservation and steam engines. The term entered the food world around 1890, when the USDA (United States Department of Agriculture) used the word "calorie" for a report on nutrition. The calorie we now see written on nutrition labels is the amount of heat needed to raise 1 kilogram of water by 1°C.But Here there is a problem: Your body isn't a steam engine. Unlike steam engine running on heat, your body runs on chemical energy, fueled by the oxidation of carbohydrates, fats, and protein that occurs in your cells' mitochondria. "You could say mitochondria are like small power plants," says Maciej Buchowski, PhD, a research professor of medicine at Vanderbilt University Medical Center. "Instead of one central plant, you have several billion on each cell, so it's more efficient." Your move: Track carbohydrates, fats, and protein—not just calories—when you're evaluating foods.

3) Eat Water Filled Foods :

Foods with a high water content—think soups, salads, cucumbers and watermelon—help you feel full and satisfied on fewer calories. (Interestingly, drinking water alongside foods doesn't have the same effect. Starting your meal with a broth-based soup or salad (not drenched in dressing) may help you eat less of your main course. A recent weight-loss trial showed that dieters who drank 2 cups of water before eating lost more weight than those who didn't.

Water is an important need of our body as it is 70% comprised of water and also, many of the vitamins and minerals we need are water-soluble and they are also absorbed better when in solution.

Amazingly, it is not only a glass of water which can only fulfill our liquid needs rather this world is full of natural foods which are rich in water content and hence, could be used to keep the water level balanced in our bodies and could contribute towards healthy life in this way.

Water rich foods are mostly comprised of vegetables and fruits which do not only contain anti-oxidants but are also alkalizing. This, in turn, minimizes acidity in our body and also contributes towards better joints, bones and tissue repair. Moreover, water rich food items establApart from that, water rich foods are really useful in losing weight and fighting ageing as such foods are high in silica giving skin tissue, collagen and elastin a boost, which means less wrinkling and stronger muscles. Moreover, these water-rich foods are low in calories which mean you can eat a good amount of them without even feeling guilty or scared about putting up weight.

All in all, it is very beneficial to have water rich fruits and vegetables in one's diet. We shall now look at the top water rich foods in the below section-

a) Crisp Lettuce- Crisp lettuce contains 96% water within itself. Hence, it helps a lot in keeping up with the hydration needs of your body. Apart from that it is also a good source of potassium, antioxidants and smaller amounts of vitamins C and K. So if you are looking up for water rich foods then crisp lettuce is a must-try. You can use it in your salad on routine basis.

b) Watermelon- Watermelon is not only refreshing and tasty rather it is enriched with a lot of water content, you can find 91% water in it along with a good amount of vitamins A and C. moreover, it also contains lycopene, fiber and potassium. In other words, it is the best fruit which you can opt out for to fulfill the water needs of your body as it gives you a win-win situation.ish a system in our bodies that detoxes itself efficiently.

c) Grape Fruit- Grape fruit has 90% water content and hence, comes on 3rd spot in our list. It is also low in terms of calories and is considered as a good source of phytonutrients and vitamin C. So this is another lucrative option which can provide you with good amount of energy and hydration.

d) Broccoli- Broccoli is very commonly used vegetable in west but do you know it contains almost 89 percent water. In addition, it includes vitamin C, calcium, fiber, iron and beta carotene which later, gets converted into vitamin A by body. Therefore, it is very beneficial for you to eat as much broccoli as possible because it makes your body water-rich.

e) Low-Fat Milk and Yogurt- Low fat milk and yogurt contains 89% and 85% water content respectively and hence, it comes on 5th position in this list. This food qualifies as a good source to add protein, phosphorus, potassium and vitamins A and D to your diet. So, what are you waiting for? Go and have them today.

f) Coconut Water- Coconut water is comprised of 95 percent water. It is commonly found in coconut that is how it differs from coconut milk. It is a good choice for sportsperson to keep their bodies hydrated as it has relatively low carbohydrate and low sodium content.

g) Avocado- Avocado contains 81% water as well as many other health fats which are very beneficial for the body. Moreover, absorption of two key carotenoids, lycopene and beta-carotene also increased by 200 to 400 percent when fresh avocados was added to meals. It is very good to speed up the recovery process in athletes as well.

h) Cucumbers- Cucumbers have 96 percent water content and a good balance of electrolytes for instance, calcium, magnesium, potassium and sodium. Apart from that you can also find, other potent minerals and silica which are very useful for connective tissue such as muscles, tendons, ligaments, cartilage and bone.

i) Strawberries- Strawberry is another very good water rich fruit as it contains 92% of water content as well as only 23 calories. Moreover, strawberries also speed up and regulate the blood sugar response in individuals due to the polyphenols found in them.

j) Celery- Celery is also full of water content and can be made a part of your daily water-rich diet. In fact celery is a very effective and powerful electrolyte food as two to three mineral-rich stalks of celery can refill sodium, potassium, magnesium, calcium, phosphorus, iron and zinc levels in athletes after intense exercise. So if you are a sportsperson then this is what you want to keep yourself hydrated and full of all the required minerals.

4) They Drink Tea Every Morning! :

"I always start with ginger tea, which is a black tea with milk, honey, ginger, and cardamom," Top Chef host Padma Lakshmi , about her breakfast ritual. "Then I'll have a green juice with kale, beets, mint, apple, carrots, and ginger or a three-egg-white, one-yolk scramble. If I'm hungry, I'll add half a cup of 1 percent cottage cheese to the eggs." We love tea so much, we made it part of our bestselling new diet plan, The 7-Day Flat-Belly Tea Cleanse! Test panelists lost up to 4 inches from their waist!

5) They Divide And Dine :

Until all restaurants become BYOP (bring your own plate), you'll need to shrink your serving in a different way: When your plate of foods arrives, dive in and eat half, then wait at least 10 minutes before Starting round 2.While you are waiting at least 10 minutes before Starting round 2, you chat and sip water, and your stomach will have a chance to digest and decide whether you've had enough ,and whether you really want to start round 2 or not — no matter what the plate's saying.

6) They just want to be satisfied , than be stuffed with food :

On a fullness scale of 1 to 10, skinny women stop eating at a level of 6 or 7, says Jill Fleming, author of "Thin People Don't Clean Their Plates." The rest of us not so thin people may keep eating until 8 or 10. Why? It Is because you mistakenly equate the sensation of fullness with satisfaction and feel deprived if you stop short, says Fleming. And also you are used to finishing what's in front of you, regardless of whether you really need it.Well,good old mama taught you to always clean the plates, which might not be good for your waistline ,and your health. To eat like Thin People, about halfway through your next meal, put your spoon down and, using the fullness scale of 1 to 10, rate your level of fullness. Do it again when you have about some food left. The goal here is to get into the habit of leaving some food on the plate everytime you eat, and it also helps you to increase your awareness of how satisfied you feel during a meal. Rating your level of fullness while you are eating ,also helps to slows down your eating, which also allows the feelings of fullness to settle in.

7) They Know hunger is not really an emergency :

Most of us who struggle with extra pounds tend to view hunger as a "emegency situation" that needs to be solved—and fast, says Judith S. Beck, PhD, author of " The New Beck Diet Solution. " If you fear hunger, you might routinely over-eat to avoid hunger," she says. Thin people tolerate hunger because they know that feelings of hunger always comes even if you just had food just 15 minutes ago, and if you just tolerate the hunger for 5 to 10 minutes or so, you will find that ,surprisingly, you are not that hungry anymore. Fear and Hunger are interconnected,just like Fear and Money are interconnected.When you don't have enough Money, you are in Fear that You will loose your House,you will loose your family,your children,God! You will everything! cause everything needs Money to buy! Including you will loose your own life,if you can't pay the debt. So,Fear and Hunger is very similar to Fear and Money, because when you are in Hunger, the voice inside you is telling you that you are going to die, you will loose your life, there is not enough food to keep you alive! That voice inside of you is a voice who was alive since millions of years ago, that voice was living alongside your great great great grandfather when they were living in the African Safari where today at this moment in the African Safari,animals are literally eating one another ,just so they can stay alive.Did you see on the Youtube on Africa Safari, where the Hyenas were constantly trying to snatch the food away from the lioness,say, a buffallo killed by the lioness? The situation is so dire that the hyenas is willing to risk its life everyday to snatch the food. So this dire situation is the normal situation from millions of year until now.When I say until now, I do not mean that we the world have solve the food situation today. In fact, millions of people are in hunger every single day, despite the so-called "Progress" we have made.We might be using computers and travelling on an airplanes, but the problem of money supply,or in other words, the lack of money has not been solved. So why despite all of the material progress, the money supply has still not been solve? Don't know. So the point here is that "Fear And Hunger" are interlink in so many ways.You are hungry? You don't look that very thin? Maybe you have money problem? maybe you have family problems?or any relationships problems? Maybe you are afraid of loosing your job, your house? everything? Try The Pick-a- busy-day to purposely delay lunch by an hour or two. Or try skipping an afternoon snack . You'll see that you can skip all those meals, and still function just fine. The next time you feel those grumbles, you'll hold off before making a beeline for the fridge.

8) Imagine Eating Before You Eat :

Picture this: someone in your office brings in doughnuts and places them where you can't miss them. But before grabbing one as you pass by, you stop, close your eyes and imagine you| eating the doughnut...slowly. Sure, your co-workers might think you're a little weird, but there's a good chance that doing this will keep you from eating as much as you would otherwise. A recent study in Science found that people presented M&Ms who first imagined eating 30 of them one at a time ate fewer of the candies than those who dove right in without the visualization exercise. Researchers think that the repeated imagining got subjects used to the food, which made them crave it less. Or it could just be that if you put that much thought into what you're about to eat, you pretty much safeguard yourself against mindless eating.

9) Thin People eat more fruits :

Skinny women, on average, have one more serving of fruit and eat more fiber and less fat per day than overweight people, reports a 2006 study published in the Journal of the American Dietetic Association.Start tinkering. To eat like a skinny women, examine your diet for ways to add whole fruits (not juices) to your meals and snacks. Aim for two or three servings per day. Sprinkle berries in your cereal or on your yogurt. Add sliced pears to your turkey sandwich, or bake an apple for dessert. Keep a bowl of fruit on your kitchen table or desk to motivate you to think fruit first, vending machine later or never.

10) Thin people look after themselves first :

For five years, Anne Fletcher, a registered dietitian and the author of Thin for Life (Houghton Mifflin, $15, amazon.com), worked in an obesity clinic. "So often the women I saw were people who refused to take time for themselves," she recalls. "Their whole lives were spent giving, giving, giving—which women tend to do anyway, but it was really to a fault. Sometimes you need to put yourself first."Thin women prioritize eating right, exercising regularly, and reducing stress—all of which are conducive to staying slim. Fletcher confesses to missing the occasional Little League game to work out but contends that such behavior shouldn't induce guilt. Rather, it's about taking care of yourself."When people take the reins, they realize that the solution to weight control is inside them, not in some magic potion or fad diet that their mother or sister is on.

11) Thin People Exercise :

Forty-two percent of study participants of thin people reported exercising five or more times a week. Exercise does so much for our bodies and brains, including reducing stress and depression symptoms as well as the risk of diabetes and a host of other conditions. One more really cool side effect of habitual exercise is that it'll make you crave a healthier diet. That's a win-win for weight loss. The endorphin rush you get from a sprint around the neighborhood might help you resist temptation, whether that's alcohol or a big slice of chocolate cake.

12) Thin People eat mindfully :

People who look and feel good generally don't put themselves on restrictive diets. Instead, they think about what they're putting in their bodies. While 74 percent said they never or rarely diet, 92 percent reported being conscious of what they ate. This number suggests that effortlessly slim people don't engage in mindless eating or eating out of boredom or with a purpose beyond addressing hunger. As it seems, naturally thin people are naturally thin in part because they don't make thinness their main priority. They take a "be" not "do" approach, incorporating healthy habits into their routines on the regular. If you want to follow suit, a lifestyle shift may be in order.

13) Thin People are creatures of habit :

Any dietitian will tell you that a varied diet is good--but too much variety can backfire, says Katz, author of The Flavor Point Diet. Studies have shown that too many tastes and textures encourage you to overeat, he explains. "Thin people have what I call a food groove— the majority of their meals consist of well-planned staples," says

Beck. "There are a few surprises thrown in, but for the most part, their diets are fairly predictable."Try to eat as consistently as possible with your major meals—have cereal for breakfast, a salad at lunch, and so forth. It's okay to add grilled chicken to the salad one day and tuna the next, but by sticking to a loosely prescribed meal schedule, you limit the opportunities to overindulge.

14) Thin People have a Scale :

Thin people have scale to weight themselves.About 50 percent said they weighed themselves at least once a week. New research finds that weighing yourself daily is a good habit for losing weight and maintaining a healthy size. "Stepping on the scales should be like brushing your teeth," David Levitsky, a professor of nutrition and psychology at Cornell University.While the number on a scale is only one way to weight loss, it can indicate a progress toward a healthy lifestyle. That said, weighing habits can be problematic for certain individuals. For some, weighing themselves can cause depression and stress and even counterproductive behavior like emotional eating. The feeling of defeat when reading a number may also override successes. If you sense that the scale does you more harm than good, skip this tip.

15)Thin People Don't waste time on diet foods :

Foods with low-fat or low-calorie labels sound good in theory. The problem is that these are often heavily processed and high in carbs. "These will convert to sugar in your body, potentially contributing to weight gain," says Heiser. What's more, companies enhance these products after removing fat by pumping them with sugar, salt and other additives. "Women who don't diet are still reading ingredient labels," says Lori Shemek, PhD, author of the forthcoming book Fight FATflammation. But they do that to cut through the tricky health claims splashed across the front of the package to find out what's really in the food.

16) No food is "bad." :

It doesn't pay to refer to brownies as "bad" and kale as "good." In a University of Toronto study, women who were deprived of chocolate for a week experienced more cravings and were more likely to eat more chocolate. A later 2010 study confirmed the results: If you tell yourself you can't have chocolate and try not to think about chocolate, you obsess over...chocolate. And find yourself scarfing Snickers. It ties back to thinking you're a dieting failure, which makes you feel guilty and overeat as a result. For a happier relationship with food, ditch "bad" from your vocabulary.

Bad' Foods Can Help You Lose Fat-Seductive foods seem to lurk at every turn, especially when you're trying to lose weight. But many foods that have gotten a bad rap aren't so terrible after all. Learn which tempting treats can actually help you lose weight and keep it off.

a) Eggs- When it comes to healthy eating, few foods have sparked as much debate as eggs. The latest research suggests an egg a day is safe and nutritious for most adults -- and if you eat that egg for breakfast, you'll boost your odds of losing weight. The reason: Eggs are packed with protein, which takes time to digest. Eating protein in the morning keeps your stomach full, so you eat less during the rest of the day.

b) Steak- For years, health experts have been admonishing us to eat less red meat. But steak is not always bad for the waistline. In fact, a lean cut of beef has barely more saturated fat than a similar-sized skinless chicken breast. Like eggs, steak is loaded with protein and can keep you feeling full longer. To get plenty of protein with less fat, choose tenderloin, sirloin, or other extra-lean cuts -- and limit portions to the size of your palm.

c) Pork- Talk about a bad reputation -- the term "pork" is used to describe all kinds of excess, so it's no wonder dieters often steer clear. Here's a case where the meat itself is not what it used to be.

Today's cuts of pork tenderloin are 31% leaner than 20 years ago. That makes this white meat a lean source of protein with benefits similar to those of lean beef.

d) Pasta- Rather than avoiding pasta when you're dieting, make the switch to whole grain and keep your portions small. Research suggests people who eat several servings of whole-grain foods per day are more likely to slim down and maintain healthy weights. According to one study, eating whole grains rather than refined grains can also help burn belly fat.

e) Nuts- Nuts may be high in fat, but it's the good kind. And they are also rich in nutrients, protein, and fiber, which can help stabilize blood sugar. Sure, you'll get a few extra grams of fat from munching on a handful of nuts, but it's worth it if it helps you avoid reaching for cookies or other sweets. Even peanut butter can be a dieter's friend. In one study people who ate a handful of nuts a day were slimmer and even lived longer.

f) Cheese- Dieters often try to cut calories by nixing calcium-rich dairy foods, but some studies suggest this is a mistake. One theory is that the body burns more fat when it gets enough calcium, so eating low-fat cheese, yogurt, and milk may actually contribute to weight loss. Calcium supplements don't seem to yield the same benefits, so a diet rich in dairy may have other factors at work as well. Dairy foods are also rich in protein, which helps keep you feeling full.

g) Coffee--Coffee only falls in the "bad" category when you drink too much of it (3-5 cups a day) or mix in cream, sugar, or flavored syrups. Drink it black without added fat and calories. Drink it skinny: Stir in skim milk for added calcium and vitamin D, and artificial sweetener or one teaspoon of sugar.

Bad Foods -- Good Portions- Just about any "bad" food can be part of your weight loss plan if you stick to small enough portions. In fact, dietitians advise against banning your favorite treats. Depriving yourself of the foods you crave could set you up for failure. A better strategy is to set limits on quantity -- for example, one chocolate truffle a day -- and stick to them.

17)Thin People Step Away From the Screen :

One of our favorite things about lunchtime is that it gives us a break from our desks. And stepping away from the computer during lunch has an added health bonus, according to recent research in the American Journal of Clinical Nutrition: it may help you eat less. Participants in the study either ate lunch while playing solitaire on a computer or ate without any distractions (no computer). When quizzed on their feelings of fullness 30 minutes later, the undistracted eaters reported feeling fuller than the group that ate in front of a computerscreen. Not only that, when they snacked later on, they ate less.

18) An Apple a Day Melts the Pounds Away! :

Apples are packed with fiber and water, so your stomach will want less. Plus, studies out of Washington State and Brazil have shown that people who eat at least three apples or pears a day lose weight. Here's how it works: All you have to do to get started is to add healthier choices to whatever else you're already eating. Before you dig into whatever it is you really want to eat, have something with some natural fiber in it — ideally, an apple — because in all the medical literature, the one dietary component most associated with weight loss is fiber consumption. The reason fiber helps us control our weight is that it fills the belly yet yields few calories since fiber is, for the most part, not something that we can digest. It also slows down the digestion of food, so you get a slow and steady source of glucose sans the rollercoaster ride of blood sugar crazies and the cravings that follow.And apples don't have just any old fiber, they are a rich source of a particularly powerful kind called pectin. It's what's used as a gelling agent to make jams and jellies, and in our stomach it can delay stomach emptying through a similar mechanism. Researchers at UCLA showed that by swapping in pectin for regular fiber, they could double the time it took subjects' stomachs to empty from about 1 hour to 2 hours, which meant subjects felt full that much longer.[1] And in another study published in the journal Nutrition, scientists found that instructing participants to eat an apple or a pear before meals resulted in significant weight loss.[2]

19) Persistence is the key :

Losing weight and then not able to keep it off of your body does not sound good at all and unfortunately, most of the time, the same thing happens especially when you follow crush diets, supplements that are quick in their results but the effects are not long lasting, you happen to use remedies that surely show results but may cause some side effects too.Slimming body should be your goal but neglecting health should not be even an option as good health is mandatory.Do remember, people who lose a huge amount of weight are only able to achieve the large weight loss because they understand that the steady and slowly they progress, the better the chances of losing weight will be.Strong will power and being persistent is the right Mantra to lose weight.Because the short cuts may work for you but they will not be capable of providing you the long lasting results and when you are willing to embrace a healthy life style then why don't you adapt it for good rather just for a mere period of 6 month or 1 to 2 years.

20) Thin people don't sit still :

On average, skinny women are on their feet an extra 2 1/2 hours per day—which can help burn off 33 pounds a year, according to a study from the Mayo Clinic in Rochester, MN.Try a reality check. Studies have shown that people often overestimate how active they really are, says Gallagher. Most people actually spend 16 to 20 hours a day just sitting. Wear a pedometer on an average day, and see how close you get to the recommended 10,000 steps. Your day should combine 30 minutes of structured exercise with a variety of healthy habits, such as taking the stairs instead of the elevator or mopping the floor with extra vigor. At the Endocrine Research Unit of the Mayo Clinic, in Rochester, Minnesota, a study of 20 self-proclaimed couch potatoes—half of whom were lean, half mildly obese—revealed that the thin volunteers were more likely to stand, walk, and fidget. The researchers noted that the obese participants sat, on average, more than two hours longer every day than the lean ones did."If the obese subjects took on the activity levels of the lean volunteers, they could burn through about 350 calories more a day without working out," says endocrinologist James Levine, the lead author of the study. "Over a year, this alone could result in a weight loss of approximately 30 pounds, if calorie intake remained the same."Simply moving around more, taking walks during the workday, and parking your car at the far end of the parking lot can burn many calories. But regular exercise is important, too. "Ninety percent of people who maintain their weight are exercising in a way that's the equivalent of walking four miles a day," says registered dietitian Elizabeth Somer, the author of 10 Habits That Mess Up a Woman's Diet (McGraw-Hill, $17, amazon.com).Johnson, for instance, does "some yoga stretching and light weights in the morning." Then, she says, "I combine a run with walking my son to the bus. I'll usually get some aerobic exercise every day."Regular workouts have another dividend: "Exercise makes you more aware of your body," psychologist Stephen Gullo says. "You're less likely to eat the chocolate cake that you know will take hours to burn off on the treadmill."

21) Thin people live Outdoor :

OK, So thin people does not exactly live outdoor,but they go out more often. Thin people value outdoor living and health and wellness more," says James O. Hill, Ph.D., director of the Center for Human Nutrition at the University of Colorado Health Sciences Center, in Denver, who has lived there for 14 years. "People will take off every Friday because they go to the mountains. They're willing to prioritize health and wellness."Its no accident that Colorado has fewer fat people .The state has the country's largest system of city parks, more than 3 million acres of national parks and forests, 10 major ski resorts, and 400 mountain-biking trails. In addition, 20 percent of Coloradans belong to health clubs—the second-highest percentage in the United States. (Delaware has the highest.) Colorado's weather also helps. Says Hill: "We have 300-plus days each year when it's nice to be outside."

22) Thin People take the stairs rather than the elevators to cut calories :

Taking the stairs for a total of just two minutes, five days a week, gives you the same calorie-burning results as a 20-minute walk.Stair climbing is an excellent exercise to burn calories that anyone can do to naturally speed up their metabolism getting places. The only reason you should be taking the elevator is if the stairs are down. You don't need a stair climber to climb stairs, do it for real. Just minutes a day can turn into tens and hundreds of calories burnt off not to mention the strength building it does for your legs.In Japan there is a diet and weight-loss method called the staircase diet that to no surprise helps you burn calories just by going up and down stairs. For most people the task of climbing stairs is a rudimentary task something almost second nature as walking. On the other hand, the other half of us who ride the elevator hoping the power doesn't go out are missing out.There is a Japanese proverb that goes something like this. Even pebbles can become a mountain. Moreover, in terms of your diet, simple stair climbing can turn into climbing mountains. The minutes you speed in getting around each day makes a big difference in maintaining weight and climbing stairs is just as respectable as any other self-proclaimed exercise routine.

23) Add fun activities :

Spend even just half an hour tossing a ball or Frisbee with your kid.Tossing a Frisbee. Hitting the dance floor. Crushing your friend in Wii tennis. They're all great ways to pass the time and let off some steam, but it turns out that some of your favorite hobbies might qualify as actual exercise too.Even light physical activities—things you view as more fun and leisurely than "fitness"—can reduce stress, punch up your metabolism, and add years to your life. They can also help speed up recovery from traditional workouts and ease sore muscles.Now, don't go canceling your trainer just yet: Eighteen holes of mini golf or tug-of-war with your pooch doesn't necessarily match the muscle-building, fat-blasting potential of a 20-minute strength workout.

a) Frisbee Toss - DEPENDS. A little back-and-forth won't burn a ton of cals, but a competitive session will.Ultimate Frisbee leagues have sprung up across the country (find one near you at usaultimate.org); players dive, jump, and pass the disk into an end zone. It's a great workout, says Melissa Witmer, founder of Ultimate Results in Lancaster, Pennsylvania. You don't need to join a team; use Ultimate Frisbee as inspiration and send your bud tough-to-catch leading passes.kout. But there may be ways to turn these fun exercises into a genuine sweat session.

b) Fetch With Fido - FUN. Your dog is the one running after the ball, right? If you just stand and wait, even a big throw doesn't amount to much.While research suggests that pet owners get more exercise than those without pets, the exercise is typically consistent and active, like daily walks. But ball tossing can benefit you too, if you get yourself in the game, says Jill Bowers, a personal (and dog) trainer at Thank Dog! Bootcamp in Los Angeles. Carry a toy or stick and run, shuffle, or backpedal with your dog in tow, changing movements every 30 seconds. After one minute, launch the toy and bang out five pushups before your dog brings it back.

c) Virtual Sports - FITNESS. No joke, some video games can actually sub for a decent workout. The top games use your whole body to control on-screen movement, says Elizabeth DiRico, an exercise physiologist and author of a 2009 study on active video games. "Choose ones that have you punching, swinging, squatting, or moving side to side," she says. According to another study on Wii sport games, boxing demanded the most effort, with baseball and tennis ranking as moderate activity. Buddy up for bonus points: Playing with someone in the room can prompt you to work harder than you would with a virtual competitor.

d) Soccer Burns More Fat Than Jogging - A new scientific experiment shows that soccer is better for your health than jogging. Researchers believe that soccer can be used to actively fight obesity. Soccer is not just a game of fun. The research shows that a game of soccer two to three times a week is profoundly health-improving. As a matter of fact, the beneficial effects are so massive that it beats jogging.Sports scientist Peter Krustrup and his colleagues from the University of Copenhagen, the Copenhagen University Hospital and Bispebjerg Hospital have followed a soccer team consisting of 14 untrained men aged 20 to 40 years.For a period of 3 months, the players have been subjected to a number of tests such as fitness ratings, total mass of muscles, percentage of fat, blood pressure, insulin sensitivity and balance.

Surprising results - 2-3 weekly rounds of soccer practise, of the duration of app. 1 hour, released massive health and training benefits. Their percentage of fat went down, the total mass of muscle went up, their blood pressure fell and their fitness ratings improved significantly. Everything we tested improved, says Peter Krustrup.In parallel with the soccer-experiment, the research group did the same tests on a group of joggers as well as on a passive control group. The joggers also trained 2-3 times a week, but their efforts showed smaller effect than that of the soccer players.

CHAPTER 2

24) Take a Multivitamin :

There's no magic pill for weight loss, but taking a daily multivitamin may help you shed pounds. In a study of more than 85 obese women in India, those who took a multivitamin (with 29 vitamins and minerals, much like a "one-a-day" you find on store shelves), while continuing to eat their normal diets, lost an average of three and a half pounds over six months. Those who took a placebo lost nothing. The findings, published in the International Journal of Obesity, add to a growing field of research that connects vitamins and minerals to weight loss. One plausible theory as to why multivitamins might help in weight loss, advice Angelo Tremblay, Ph.D., an obesity researcher at Laval University in Quebec City, is that when your body is low on vitamins and minerals, your appetite fires up—prompting you to eat more to replenish the nutrients you're missing. By staying topped off with nutrients, on the other hand, it is possible to keep a uncontrollable appetite under control.

25)DEPRESSION AND WEIGHT GAIN:

a) **Depression Leads to Weight Gain, Study Confirms-** A new study at the University of Alabama at Birmingham (UAB) confirms the relationship between depression and abdominal obesity, which has been linked to an increased risk for cancer and cardiovascular disease."We found that in a sample of young adults during a 15-year period, those who started out reporting high levels of depression gained weight at a faster rate than others in the study, but starting out overweight did not lead to changes in depression," said UAB Assistant Professor of Sociology Belinda Needham, PhD. The study appears in the June issue of the American Journal of Public Health.

"Our study is important because if you are interested in controlling obesity, and ultimately eliminating the risk of obesity-related diseases, then it makes sense to treat people's depression," said Needham, who teaches in the UAB department of sociology and social work. "It's another reason to take depression seriously and not to think about it just in terms of mental health, but to also think about the physical consequences of mental health problems."

Needham examined data from the Coronary Artery Risk Development in Young Adults (CARDIA) study, a longitudinal study of 5,115 men and women ages 18-30 that aimed to identify the precursors of cardiovascular disease. Needham studied the data to test whether body mass index (BMI) — weight divided by the square of one's height — and waist circumference were associated with increases in depression or whether depression was associated with changes in BMI and waist circumference during a period of time.

b) Coping with Depression - Depression suck out your energy, hope, and ambitions, making it difficult to take the steps that will help you to feel better. But while overcoming depression isn't quick or easy, it's not impossible. You can't just condition yourself to "snap out of it," but you do have more control than you realize—even if your depression is severe and persistent. The main thing is to start small and go from there. Feeling better takes time, but you can get there by making positive choices for yourself each day.

Dealing with depression requires action, but taking action when you're depressed can be hard. Sometimes, just thinking about the things you should do to feel better, like exercising or spending time with family, can seem exhausting or impossible to put into action.

Depression recovery is a catch -22: The stuff which help the most are the things that are the hardest to do. There is a big difference, however, between something that's hard and something that's impossible. You may not have much energy, but by drawing on all your reserves, you should have enough to take a walk around the block or pick up the phone to call a friend.Taking the first step is always the hardest. But going for a walk or getting up and dancing to your favorite music, for example, is something you can do immediately. And it can significantly boost your mood and energy for several hours—long enough to put a second recovery step into action, such as preparing a mood-boosting meal or arranging to meet an old friend. By taking the following small but progressive steps day in a day out, you'll soon lift the heavy burden of depression and find yourself feeling happier, healthier, and more drive again.Support plays an important role in overcoming depression. On your own, it can be difficult to maintain a positive views of life and maintain the effort required to beat depression. At the same time, the very nature of depression makes it difficult to ask for help. When you're depressed, the tendency is to withdraw and isolate so that connecting to even close family members and friends can be hard.

You may feel too tired to talk,ashamed at your situation, or feels guilty of certain relationships. But this is just the depression's projection of action. Staying connected to other people and taking part in social activities will make a world of difference in your mood and outlook. Reaching out is not a sign of weakness and it won't mean you're an embarrasment to others. Your loved ones care about you and want to helps you. And if you don't feel that you have anyone to turn to, it's never too late to create new relationships thus improving your support networK.

c) **How to reach out for support to deal with your depression -** Find support from people who make you feel better. The person you talk to doesn't have to be able to fix you,they just need to be a good listener—someone who will listen attentively and compassionately without being distracted or judging you.Phone calls, social media, and texting are great ways to stay in touch, but they don't replace good old-fashioned in-person quality time. The simple act of talking to someone face to face about how you feel can play a big role in relieving depression and keeping it away.Try to keep up with social communication even if you don't feel like it. Often when you're depressed, it feels more comfortable to retreat into yourself, but being with people will make you feel less depressed.Find ways to support others. It's nice to receive support, but research shows you get an even bigger mood boost from providing support yourself. So find ways—both big and small—to help others: volunteer, be a listening ear for a friend, do something nice for somebody.Care for a pet. While nothing can replace the human connection, pets can bring joy and companionship into your life and help you feel less isolated. Caring for a pet can also get you outside of yourself and give you a sense of being needed—both powerful antidotes to depression.

Join a support group for depression. Being with others dealing with depression can go a long way in reducing your sense of isolation. You can also encourage each other, give and receive advice on how to cope, and share your experiences.

d) Tips for staying connected -

i) Take a class or join a club or some association

ii) Have conversation with a friend

iii) communicate with a teacher, coach or motivator

iv) Talk to one person about your feelings

v) Have lunch or coffee with a friend

vi) Ask someone you trust to check in with you regularly

vii) Go for a walk with someone

e) Do things that you like- Do things that give you relaxation and energy . This includes following a healthy lifestyle, learning how to better manage stress, setting limits on what you're able to do, and scheduling fun activities into your day.While you can't force yourself to have fun or experience pleasure, you can push yourself to do things, even when you don't feel like it. You might be surprised at how much better you feel once you're out in the world. Even if your depression doesn't lift immediately, you'll gradually feel more upbeat and energetic as you make time for fun activities.

i) Play some sports you like, soccer,basket ball, cricket,volley ball.

ii) Go to the Zoo,watching all the animals in their natural habitate will reminds you of how humans used to live,that realization will makes you happy.

f) Look after your health - Get enough sleep. Depression is linked to sleep situation, be it whether you are having too much or too little sleep, your mood goes up and down. Get on a healthy sleep schedule by learning healthy sleep habits.Always keep in check of your stress. stress cause depression. Figure out all the things in your life that give you stress, such as over-work, money problems, or negative relationships, and find ways to fix the negative situation and regain control.

26) Develop different kind of ways to deal with depression:

a) Think of a list of things that you can do to fix your mood situation. The more ways for coping with depression, the better. Use a few of these different ways each day.

b) Use "mother nature" to fix you depression.

c) Go to the library to get a good book to read.

d) Watch a interesting movie,one that you like

e) Do something out of the box

f) Have a good shower for yourself

g) Think about what you like about yourself

h) Play with your dog,or get pet snake,or pet crow,or pet dolphin.

i) Have conversation with someone without the help of any electronics.

When you're depressed, just getting out of bed can seem like a daunting task, let alone working out! But exercise is a powerful depression fighter—and one of the most important tools in your recovery arsenal. Research shows that regular exercise can be as effective as medication for relieving depression symptoms. It also helps prevent relapse once you're well.To get the most benefit, aim for at least 30 minutes of exercise per day. This doesn't have to be all at once—and it's okay to start small. A 10-minute walk can improve your mood for two hours.

27)Exercise is something you can do right now to boost your mood:

Your fatigue will improve if you stick with it. Starting to exercise can be difficult when you're depressed and feeling exhausted. But research shows that your energy levels will improve if you keep with it. Exercise will help you to feel energized and less fatigued, not more.Find exercises that are continuous and rhythmic. The most benefits for depression come from rhythmic exercise—such as walking, weight training, swimming, martial arts, or dancing—where you move both your arms and legs.Add a mindfulness element, especially if your depression is rooted in unresolved trauma or fed by obsessive, negative thoughts. Focus on how your body feels as you move—such as the sensation of your feet hitting the ground, or the feeling of the wind on your skin, or the rhythm of your breathing.Pair up with an exercise partner. Not only does working out with others enable you to spend time socializing, it can also help to keep you motivated. Try joining a running club, taking a water aerobics or dance class, seeking out tennis partners, or enrolling in a soccer or volleyball league.Take a dog for a walk. If don't own a dog, you can volunteer to walk homeless dogs for an animal shelter or rescue group. You'll not only be helping yourself but also be helping to socialize and exercise the dogs, making them more adoptable.

28) Eat a healthy, depression-fighting diet :

What you eat has a direct impact on the way you feel. Reduce your intake of foods that can adversely affect your brain and mood, such as caffeine, alcohol, trans fats, and foods with high levels of chemical preservatives or hormones (such as certain meats).Don't skip meals. Going too long between meals can make you feel irritable and tired, so aim to eat something at least every three to four hours.Minimize sugar and refined carbs. You may crave sugary snacks, baked goods, or comfort foods such as pasta or French fries, but these "feel-good" foods quickly lead to a crash in mood and energy. Aim to cut out as much of these foods as possible.Boost your B vitamins. Deficiencies in B vitamins such as folic acid and B-12 can trigger depression. To get more, take a B-complex vitamin supplement or eat more citrus fruit, leafy greens, beans, chicken, and eggs.Boost your mood with foods rich in omega-3 fatty acids. Omega-3 fatty acids play an essential role in stabilizing mood. The best sources are fatty fish such as salmon, herring, mackerel, anchovies, sardines, tuna, and some cold-water fish oil supplements.

29) Get a daily dose of sunlight :

Sunlight can help boost serotonin levels and improve your mood. Whenever possible, get outside during daylight hours and expose yourself to the sun for at least 15 minutes a day. Remove sunglasses (but never stare directly at the sun) and use sunscreen as needed.Take a walk on your lunch break, have your coffee outside, enjoy an al fresco meal, or spend time gardening.Double up on the benefits of sunlight by exercising outside. Try hiking, walking in a local park, or playing golf or tennis with a friend.Increase the amount of natural light in your home and workplace by opening blinds and drapes and sitting near windows.If you live somewhere with little winter sunshine, try using a light therapy box.

30) Dealing with the winter blues :

For some people, the reduced daylight hours of winter lead to a form of depression known as seasonal affective disorder (SAD). SAD can make you feel like a completely different person to who you are in the summer: hopeless, sad, tense, or stressed, with no interest in friends or activities you normally love. No matter how hopeless you feel, though, there are plenty of things you can do to keep your mood stable throughout the year. See Seasonal Affective Disorder.

31) Challenge negative thinking :

Do you feel like you're powerless or weak? That bad things happen and there's not much you can do about it? That your situation is hopeless? Depression puts a negative spin on everything, including the way you see yourself and your expectations for the future.When these types of thoughts overwhelm you, it's important to remember that this is a symptom of your depression and these irrational, pessimistic attitudes—known as cognitive distortions—aren't realistic. When you really examine them they don't hold up. But even so, they can be tough to give up. You can't break out of this pessimistic mind frame by telling yourself to "just think positive." Often, it's part of a lifelong pattern of thinking that's become so automatic you're not even completely aware of it. Rather, the trick is to identify the type of negative thoughts that are fueling your depression, and replace them with a more balanced way of thinking.Negative, unrealistic ways of thinking that fuel depressionAll-or-nothing thinking – Looking at things in black-or-white categories, with no middle ground ("If I fall short of perfection, I'm a total failure.")Overgeneralization – Generalizing from a single negative experience, expecting it to hold true forever ("I can't do anything right.")

a)The mental filter – Ignoring positive events and focusing on the negative. Noticing the one thing that went wrong, rather than all the things that went right.

b) Diminishing the positive – Coming up with reasons why positive events don't count ("She said she had a good time on our date, but I think she was just being nice.")

c) Jumping to conclusions – Making negative interpretations without actual evidence. You act like a mind reader ("He must think I'm pathetic") or a fortune teller ("I'll be stuck in this dead-end job forever.")

d) Emotional reasoning – Believing that the way you feel reflects reality ("I feel like such a loser. I really am no good!")

e) 'Shoulds' and 'should-nots' – Holding yourself to a strict list of what you should and shouldn't do, and beating yourself up if you don't live up to your rules.

f) Labeling – Classifying yourself based on mistakes and perceived shortcomings ("I'm a failure; an idiot; a loser.")

32) Put your thoughts on the witness stand :

Once you identify the destructive thoughts patterns that contribute to your depression, you can start to challenge them with questions such as:

"What's the evidence that this thought is true? Not true?"

"What would I tell a friend who had this thought?"

"Is there another way of looking at the situation or an alternate explanation?"

"How might I look at this situation if I didn't have depression?"

As you cross-examine your negative thoughts, you may be surprised at how quickly they crumble. In the process, you'll develop a more balanced perspective and help to relieve your depression.

33) When to get professional help for depression :

If you've taken self-help steps and made positive lifestyle changes and still find your depression getting worse, seek professional help. Needing additional help doesn't mean you're weak. Sometimes the negative thinking in depression can make you feel like you're a lost cause, but depression can be treated and you can feel better!

Don't forget about these self-help tips, though. Even if you're receiving professional help, these tips can be part of your treatment plan, speeding your recovery and preventing depression from returning.

34) 12 Popular Weight Loss Pills and Supplements

There are many different weight loss solutions out there.This includes all sorts of pills, drugs and natural supplements.These are claimed to help you lose weight, or at least make it easier to lose weight combined with other methods.

They tend to work via one or more of these mechanisms:

Reduce appetite, making you feel more full so that you eat fewer caloriesReduce absorption of nutrients like fat, making you take in fewer caloriesIncrease fat burning, making you burn more calories

Here are the 12 popular weight loss pills and supplements, reviewed by science

a) Garcinia Cambogia Extract-

Garcinia cambogia became popular worldwide after being featured on the Dr. Oz show in 2012.It is a small, green fruit, shaped like a pumpkin.The skin of the fruit contains hydroxycitric acid (HCA). This is the active ingredient in garcinia cambogia extract, which is marketed as a diet pill.

How it works: Animal studies show that it can inhibit a fat-producing enzyme in the body and increase levels of serotonin, potentially helping to reduce cravings (1, 2).

Effectiveness: One study with 130 people compared garcinia against a dummy pill. There was no difference in weight or body fat percentage between groups (3).

A 2011 review that looked at 12 studies on garcinia cambogia found that, on average, it caused weight loss of about 2 pounds (0.88 kg) over several weeks (4).

Side effects: There are no reports of serious side effects, but some reports of mild digestive problems.

BOTTOM LINE: Even though garcinia cambogia may cause modest weight loss, the effects are so small that they probably won't even be noticeable.

b) Hydroxycut-

Hydroxycut has been around for more than a decade, and is currently one of the most popular weight loss supplements in the world.There are several different types, but the most common one is simply called "Hydroxycut."

How it works: It contains several ingredients that are claimed to help with weight loss, including caffeine and a few plant extracts.

Effectiveness: One study showed that it caused 21 lbs (9.5 kg) of weight loss over a 3 month period.

Side effects: If you are caffeine sensitive, you may experience anxiety, jitteriness, tremors, nausea, diarrhea and irritability.

BOTTOM LINE: Unfortunately, there is only one study on this supplement and no data on long-term effectiveness. More research is needed.

c) Caffeine-

Caffeine is the most commonly consumed psychoactive substance in the world (6).It is found naturally in coffee, green tea and dark chocolate, and added to many processed foods and beverages.Caffeine is a well known metabolism booster, and is often added to commercial weight loss supplements.

How it works: Short-term studies have shown that caffeine can boost metabolism by 3-11%, and increase fat burning by up to 29% (7, 8, 9, 10).

Effectiveness: There are also some studies showing that caffeine can cause modest weight loss in humans (11, 12).

Side effects: In some people, high amounts of caffeine can cause anxiety, insomnia, jitteriness, irritability, nausea, diarrhea and other symptoms. Caffeine is also addictive and can reduce the quality of your sleep.

There really is no need to take a supplement or a pill with caffeine in it. The best sources are quality coffee and green tea, which also have antioxidants and other health benefits.

BOTTOM LINE: Caffeine can boost metabolism and enhance fat burning in the short term. However, a tolerance to the effects may develop quickly.

d). Orlistat (Alli)-

Orlistat is a pharmaceutical drug, sold over-the-counter under the name Alli, and under prescription as Xenical.

How it works: This weight loss pill works by inhibiting the breakdown of fat in the gut, making you take in fewer calories from fat.

Effectiveness: According to a big review of 11 studies, orlistat can increase weight loss by 6 pounds (2.7 kg) compared to a dummy pill (13).

Other benefits: Orlistat has been shown to reduce blood pressure slightly, and reduced the risk of developing type 2 diabetes by 37% in one study (14, 15).

Side effects: This drug has many digestive side effects, including loose, oily stools, flatulence, frequent bowel movements that are hard to control, and others. It may also contribute to deficiency in fat-soluble vitamins, such as vitamins A, D, E and K.

It is usually recommended to follow a low-fat diet while taking orlistat, in order to minimize side effects.Interestingly, a low carb diet (without drugs) has been shown to be as effective as both orlistat and a low-fat diet combined (16).

BOTTOM LINE: Orlistat, also known as Alli or Xenical, can reduce the amount of fat you absorb from the diet and help you lose weight. It has many side effects, some of which are highly unpleasant.

e). Raspberry Ketones-

Raspberry ketone is a substance found in raspberries, which is responsible for their distinct smell.A synthetic version of raspberry ketones is sold as a weight loss supplement.

How it works: In isolated fat cells from rats, raspberry ketones increase breakdown of fat and increase levels of a hormone called adiponectin, believed to be related to weight loss.

Effectiveness: There is not a single study on raspberry ketones in humans, but one rat study using massive doses showed that they reduced weight gain (18).

Side effects: They may cause your burps to smell like raspberries.

BOTTOM LINE: There is no evidence that raspberry ketones cause weight loss in humans, and the rat studies showing it to work used massive doses.

f) . Green Coffee Bean Extract-

Green coffee beans are simply normal coffee beans that haven't been roasted.They contain two substances believed to help with weight loss, caffeine and chlorogenic acid.

How it works: Caffeine can increase fat burning, and chlorogenic acid can slow the breakdown of carbohydrates in the gut.

Effectiveness: Several human studies have shown that green coffee bean extract can help people lose weight (19, 20).

A review of 3 studies found that the supplement made people lose 5.4 more pounds (2.5 kg) than placebo, a dummy pill (21).

Other benefits: Green coffee bean extract may help lower blood sugar levels, and reduce blood pressure. It is also high in antioxidants (22, 23, 24, 25).

Side effects: It can cause the same side effects as caffeine. The chlorogenic acid in it may also cause diarrhea, and some people may be allergic to green coffee beans (26).

BOTTOM LINE: Green coffee bean extract may cause modest weight loss, but keep in mind that many of the studies were industry sponsored.

g) Glucomannan-

Glucomannan is a type of fiber found in the roots of the elephant yam, also called konjac.

How it works: Glucomannan absorbs water and becomes gel-like. It "sits" in your gut and promotes a feeling of fullness, helping you eat fewer calories (27).

Effectiveness: Three human studies showed that glucomannan, combined with a healthy diet, can help people lose 8-10 pounds (3.6-4.5 kg) of weight in 5 weeks (28).

Other benefits: Glucomannan is a fiber that can feed the friendly bacteria in the intestine. It can also lower blood sugar, blood cholesterol and triglycerides, and is very effective against constipation .

Side effects: It can cause bloating, flatulence and soft stools, and can interfere with some oral medications if taken at the same time.

It is important to take glucomannan about a half an hour before meals, with a glass of water.

You can find an objective review of glucomannan in this article.

BOTTOM LINE: Studies consistently show that the fiber glucomannan, when combined with a healthy diet, can help people lose weight. It also leads to improvements in various health markers.

h). Meratrim-

Meratrim is a relative newcomer on the diet pill market.It is a combination of two plant extracts that may change the metabolism of fat cells.

How it works: It is claimed to make it harder for fat cells to multiply, decrease the amount of fat that they pick up from the bloodstream, and help them burn stored fat.

Effectiveness: So far, only one study has been done on Meratrim. A total of 100 obese people were placed on a strict 2000 calorie diet, with either Meratrim or a dummy pill.

After 8 weeks, the Meratrim group had lost 11 pounds (5.2 kg) of weight and 4.7 inches (11.9 cm) off their waistlines. They also had improved quality of life and reduced blood sugar, cholesterol and triglycerides.

Side effects: No side effects have been reported.

For a detailed review of Meratrim, read this article.

BOTTOM LINE: One study showed that Meratrim caused weight loss and had a number of other health benefits. However, the study was industry sponsored and more research is needed.

i) Green Tea Extract-

Green tea extract is a popular ingredient in many weight loss supplements.This is because numerous studies have shown the main antioxidant in it, EGCG, to aid fat burning.

How it works: Green tea extract is believed to increase the activity of norepinephrine, a hormone that helps you burn fat (33).

Effectiveness: Many human studies have shown that green tea extract can increase fat burning and cause fat loss, especially in the belly area (34, 35, 36, 37).

Side effects: Green tea extract is generally well tolerated. It does contain some caffeine, and may cause symptoms in people who are caffeine sensitive.

Additionally, all of the health benefits of drinking green tea should apply to green tea extract as well.

BOTTOM LINE: Green tea and green tea extract can increase fat burning slightly, and may help you lose belly fat.

j). Conjugated Linoleic Acid (CLA)-

Conjugated linoleic acid, or CLA, has been a popular fat loss supplement for years.It is one of the "healthier" trans fats, and is found naturally in some fatty animal foods like cheese and butter.

How it works: CLA may reduce appetite, boost metabolism and stimulate the breakdown of body fat (38, 39).

Effectiveness: In a major review of 18 different studies, CLA caused weight loss of about 0.2 pounds (0.1 kg) per week, for up to 6 months (40).According to another review study from 2012, CLA can make you lose about 3 lbs (1.3 kg) of weight, compared to a dummy pill (41).

Side effects: CLA can cause various digestive side effects, and may have harmful effects over the long term, potentially contributing to fatty liver, insulin resistance and increased inflammation.

BOTTOM LINE: CLA is an effective weight loss supplement, but it may have harmful effects over the long term. The small amount of weight loss is not worth the risk.

k). Forskolin-

Forskolin is an extract from a plant in the mint family, claimed to be effective for losing weight.

How it works: It is believed to raise levels of a compound inside cells called cAMP, which may stimulate fat burning (42).

Effectiveness: One study in 30 overweight and obese men showed that forskolin reduced body fat and increased muscle mass, while having no effect on body weight. Another study in 23 overweight women found no effects (43, 44).

Side effects: There is very limited data on the safety of this supplement, or the risk of side effects.

BOTTOM LINE: The two small studies on forskolin have shown conflicting results. It is best to avoid this supplement until more research is done.

I). Bitter Orange / Synephrine-

A type of orange called bitter orange contains the compound synephrine.Synephrine is related to ephedrine, which used to be a popular ingredient in various weight loss pill formulations.However, ephedrine has since been banned as a weight loss ingredient by the FDA because of serious side effects.

How it works: Synephrine shares similar mechanisms with ephedrine, but is less potent. It can reduce appetite and significantly increase fat burning (45).

Effectiveness: Very few studies have been done on synephrine, but ephedrine has been shown to cause significant short-term weight loss in many studies (46).

Side effects: Like ephedrine, synephrine may have serious side effects related to the heart. It may also be addictive.

BOTTOM LINE: Synephrine is a fairly potent stimulant, and probably effective for weight loss in the short term. However, the side effects can be serious, so this should only be used with extreme caution.

Prescription Medication-

Additionally, there are many prescription weight loss pills that have been shown to be effective.The most common ones are Contrave, Belviq, Phentermine and Qsymia.According to a recent 2014 review study, even prescription weight loss pills don't work as well as you would hope.On average, they may help you lose up to 3-9% of body weight compared to a dummy pill .Keep in mind that this is only when combined with a healthy weight loss diet. They are ineffective on their own, and hardly a solution to obesity.Not to mention their many side effects.

Take Home Message

Out of the 12, these are the clear winners, with the strongest evidence to back them up:

Weight loss: Glucomannan, CLA and Orlistat (Alli)

Increased fat burning: Caffeine and green tea extract.However, I have to advise against Orlistat due to the unpleasant side effects, and against CLA due to the harmful effects on metabolic health.

That leaves us with glucomannan, green tea extract and caffeine.These supplements can be useful, but the effects are modest at best.Unfortunately, NO supplement or pill really works that well for weight loss.They may give your metabolism a bit of a nudge and help you lose a few pounds, but that's where it ends, unfortunately.Cutting carbs and eating more protein are still the best ways to lose weight, and work better than all the diet pills combined.

35) FASTING AND WEIGHT LOSS:

a) How Fasting At Irregular Intervals Can Help You Lose Weight-

You can loose weight in many ways.One popular ways in recently is known as irregular fasting (1).This is a way of eating that involves regular short-term fasts.Short-term fasting forced people to eat smaller portion, and also helps optimize weight control hormones.

There are different types of fastingmethods. Three popular ones are:

i. **The 16/8 Method:** Avoid having breakfast every day and eat during an 8-hour feeding window, for example, from 12 noon to 8 pm.

ii. **The 5:2 Diet:** Only consume 500-600 calories for two days of the week, but consume the other 5 days normally.

iii **Eat-Stop-Eat:** Each week,do one or two 24-hour fasting, such as not consuming dinner one day until the next dinner day.

If you do not consume too much during the periods of non-fasting, then this system will result in reduced calorie consumed and support you to lose weight and belly fat.

b) How Irregular Fasting Change Your Hormones Positively-

The body's energy is stored in body fat.When we fast, the body affect several things to make the stored energy available,which affect changes in nervous system activity, and also affect changes in several crucial hormones.Here are some of the things that change in your metabolism when you fast:

i **Insulin:** Insulin increases when we eat. When we fast, insulin decreases dramatically . Lower levels of insulin facilitate fat burning.

Ii **Human growth hormone (HGH):** Levels of growth hormone may skyrocket during a fast, increasing as much as 5-fold. Growth hormone is a hormone that can aid fat loss and muscle gain, among other things .

iii **Norepinephrine (noradrenaline):** The nervous system sends norepinephrine to the fat cells, making them break down body fat into free fatty acids that can be burned for energy.

Interestingly, despite what the 5-6 meals a day proponents would have you believe, short-term fasting may actually *increase* fat burning.Two studies have found that fasting for about 48 hours boosts metabolism by 3.6-14% . However, fasting periods that are longer can suppress metabolism.

36) Intermittent Fasting And Weight Loss:

a) Intermittent Fasting Helps You Reduce Calories and Lose Weight-

Intermittent fasting works for weight loss,because it helps you consume less.It involve skipping meals during the fasting periods. Unless you compensate by consuming much more during the ono-fasting periods, then you will be taking in fewer calories.According to a recent 2014 review study, irregular fasting can result in significant weight loss. Irregular fasting was found to reduce body weight by 3-8% in 3-24 weeks .When testing the rate of weight loss,it was found that people lost about 0.55 pounds (0.25 kg) per week with irregular fasting, but 1.65 pounds (0.75 kg) per week with alternate-day fasting.

Fasting candidate also lost 4-7% of their waist circumference, suggesting that they   lost belly fat.These results are significant, and they do show that intermittent fasting can be a useful weight loss help.All that being said, the benefits of intermittent fasting go way beyond just weight loss. It also has numerous benefits for metabolic health, and may even help prevent chronic disease and expand lifespan.Although calorie counting is generally not required when doing intermittent fasting, the weight loss is mostly mediated by an overall reduction in calorie intake.Studies comparing intermittent fasting and continuous calorie restriction show no difference in weight loss if calories are matched between groups.

BOTTOM LINE: Intermittent fasting is a helpful way to restrict calories without consciously trying to eat less. Many studies show that it can help you lose weight and belly fat.

b) Intermittent Fasting May Help You To Hold On To Your Muscle -

One of the negative effects of dieting, is that the body will burn muscle as well as fat.Interestingly, there are some studies showing that intermittent fasting may be beneficial for holding on to muscle while losing body fat.In one study, intermittent calorie denial caused a similar amount of weight loss as continuous calorie restriction, but with a much smaller reduction in muscle mass.In the calorie restriction studies, 25% of the weight lost was muscle mass, compared to only 10% in the intermittent calorie restriction studies.

One study had participants eat the same amount of calories as before, except in just one huge meal in the evening. They lost body fat and increased their muscle mass, along with a host of other beneficial changes in health markers.However, there were some limitations to these studies, so take the findings with a grain of salt.

BOTTOM LINE: There is some evidence that intermittent fasting can help you hold on to more muscle mass when dieting, compared to standard calorie restriction.

c) Irregular Fasting Encourage Healthy Eating -

One of the main benefits of Irregular fasting is the simplicity of it. I personally do the 16/8 system, in which I only consume during a certain "feeding window" every day.Instead of eating 3+ meals per day, I eat only 2, which makes it a lot easier and simpler to support my fasting lifestyle.The single best "diet" for you is the one you can stick to in the long run. If intermittent fasting makes it easier for you to stick to a   healthy diet, then this has huge benefits for long-term health and weight maintenance.

BOTTOM LINE: One of the great benefits of intermittent fasting is that it turn healthy eating simpler. This may makes it easier to keep to a healthy diet in the long term.

d)How to Succeed With an Irregular Fasting System-

There are many things you need to remember if you want to lose weight successfully by fasting :

i. **Quality of Food:** The foods you eat are very important. Try to consume mostly whole, single ingredient foods.
ii. **Calorie Count:** Calories is very important. Try to eat "normally" during the non-fasting periods, not too much that you compensate for the calories you missed when you were fasting.
iii. **Consistency:** Same as with any other weight loss system, you need to stick with it for a long period of time if you want it to be effective.
iv. **Patience:** Your body can take some time to adapt to an intermittent fasting system. Try to be consistent with your meal schedule and it will get less and less harder to fast.

Most of the popular fasting system also suggest training for strength. This is very important if you want to burn mostly body fat while holding on to muscle.In the beginning, calorie counting is generally not required with intermittent fasting. However, if your weight loss stalled, then calorie counting can be a useful tool.

BOTTOM LINE: With intermittent fasting, you still need to eat healthy and maintain a calorie deficit if you want to lose weight. Being consistent is absolutely crucial, and strength training is important.

Conclusion-

At the end of the day, intermittent fasting can be a useful tool for weight loss.This is caused primarily by consuming less, but there are also some positive effects on hormones that comes into play.Intermittent fasting is not for anyone, but can helps some people willing to do it.

37) How long can a person survive without food?

Alan D. Lieberson, a medical doctor, lawyer, and the author of Treatment of Pain and Suffering in the Terminally Ill and Advance Medical Directives, explains.The duration of survival without food is greatly influenced by factors such as body weight, genetic variation, other health considerations and, most importantly, the presence or absence of dehydration.

For total starvation in healthy individuals receiving adequate hydration, reliable data on survival are hard to obtain. At the age of 74 and already slight of build, Mahatma Gandhi, the famous nonviolent campaigner for India's independence, survived 21 days of total starvation while only allowing himself sips of water. In a 1997 article in the British Medical Journal, Michael Peel, senior medical examiner at the Medical Foundation for the Care of Victims of Torture, cites well-documented studies reporting survivals of other hunger strikers for 28, 36, 38 and 40 days. Most other reports of long-term survival of total starvation, however, have been poorly substantiated. [Editor's Note: Reports of the 1981 hunger strike by political prisoners against the British presence in Northeast Ireland indicate that 10 individuals died after periods of between 46 and 73 days without food.

Unlike total starvation, near-total starvation with continued hydration has occurred frequently, both in history and in patients under medical supervision. Survival for many months to years is common in concentration camps and during famines, but the unknown caloric intake during these times makes it impossible to predict survival. What is evident is that the body can moderate metabolism to conserve energy and that individual survival varies markedly. The body's ability to alter its metabolism is poorly understood, but it occurs at least in part through changes in thyroid function. This may help explain the evolutionary persistence of genes causing diabetes, which in the past could have allowed individuals to survive periods of starvation by enabling more economical use of energy.

Medical practitioners encounter cases of near-total starvation in patients suffering from, among other conditions, anorexia nervosa and end-stage malignancies, as well as in those following so-called starvation diets. In anorexia, death from organ failure or myocardial infarction is fairly common (up to 20 percent of cases end this way) and tends to happen when body weight has fallen to between 60 and 80 pounds (although it can occur at any time). This weight typically corresponds to a body mass index (BMI) approximately half of normal, or about 12 to 12.5. (Normal BMI is 18.5-24.9, and most fashion models have a BMI of around 17.) Unless other causes intervene, a patient with end-stage cancer often dies after losing 35 to 45 percent of his body weight. Markedly obese patients on near-starvation diets, such as those employing nutritional supplements and consuming less than 400 calories a day, may lose much more weight than that--but they start with great excesses of body fat, which can sustain metabolism. The medical community has generally rejected these diets, which were popular in the 1960s and 1970s, because participants were reportedly prone to acute myocardial infarctions.

I recall one particularly relevant experience that illustrates the inherent variability in people's ability to survive on very little food. Called in an emergency to see an out-of-town visitor with a throat abscess one Saturday afternoon, I noted his marked thinness, along with a belt showing twelve extra holes at about one-inch intervals, each showing evidence of use. I asked him about his weight and he told me he was five feet, seven inches tall and normally weighed about 145 pounds, but he thought he had noted some recent loss, maybe down to about 100 pounds over the prior year. He wasn't trying to lose weight, but it didn't bother him because he thought thinner was better. He just didn't feel like eating much. With clothes on, he weighed just 77 pounds. After he left town for further treatment, I never heard from him again, but he had seemingly lost close to half his body weight without noticing any ill effects.

In contrast to starvation with access to liquids, much more is known about survival without any sustenance (neither food nor hydration), which is a far more important practical consideration in medicine and ethics. This situation comes up frequently in two distinct medical groups--the incompetent terminally ill patients for whom artificial maintenance of life is no longer desired, and the individuals who, although not necessarily terminally ill, no longer want to live and decide to refuse food and hydration to end their lives.

A well-known example of the former is Nancy Cruzan, the subject of the famous 1990 U.S. Supreme Court decision in Cruzan versus Director, Missouri Department of Health. Cruzan was in a persistent vegetative state (PVS) for many years until she died 12 days after artificial sustenance was discontinued. Since that time, many other incidences of discontinuing sustenance in patients in a PVS have been reported and death typically occurs after 10 to 14 days. (If the individual is dehydrated or over-hydrated, the time may range from approximately one to three weeks.) In situations of voluntary refusal of food and hydration, death typically ensues on a similar time frame, although the early use of ice chips or sips of water to reduce thirst may delay this slightly.

38) How long can humans survive without food or water?

Rita Chretien, a Canadian woman survived being stranded inside a vehicle in Nevada for 48 days, by eating only some trail mix and candy, and drinking water from a stream. Apparently, she and her husband were following their GPS instructions on their way to Las Vegas from British Columbia when they took a rural road that essentially turns to a bog in the winter months. Their van eventually got stuck in the mud in the middle of nowhere, and they both waited for help for 3 days without sighting anyone. At this point, Albert Chretien, the husband, left to seek out help, while Rita remained inside the van. When she was found by a group of hunters just last week, she was nearly dead and had lost some 30lbs. Her husband remains to be found.

This recent story of near complete starvation highlights the human ability to survive for long periods of time without sustenance.

Due to obvious ethical concerns, there is not a whole lot of credible scientific data on the topic of starvation and survival. Instead, there are many accounts of either voluntary or involuntary cases of complete or near-complete starvation that allow us to make some very general conclusions.One of the most well known cases of voluntary starvation, is the hunger strike of Mahatma Ganhdi. During his protest, Gandhi ate absolutely no food and only took sips of water for 21 days, and survived. What extraordinary about this case is the fact that Gandhi was very lean when he started his hunger-strike, thus not having much energy reserve from the outset. Also, it must be noted that during his life, Gandhi is reported to have performed a total of 14 hunger strikes.

In a 1997 editorial in the British Medical Journal, Peel briefly reviewed the available literature regarding human starvation. Generally, it appears as though humans can survive without any food for 30-40 days, as long as they are properly hydrated. Severe symptoms of starvation begin around 35-40 days, and as highlighted by the hunger strikers of the Maze Prison in Belfast in the 1980s, death can occur at around 45 to 61 days.The most common cause of death in these extreme cases of starvation is myocardial infarction or organ failure, and is suggested to occur most often when a person's body mass index (BMI) reaches approximately 12.5 kg/m2.Of course, one would expect marked variability between 2 individuals in their ability to endure starvation. As suggested in a Scientific American article by

Alan Lieberson,The duration of survival without food is greatly influenced by factors such as body weight, genetic variation, other health considerations and, most importantly, the presence or absence of dehydration.I would add that body composition would also likely play a key role; for the same body weight, the individual with a greater percentage of body fat has a greater on-board storage of calories. Also, a lower muscle mass would generally be associated with reduced caloric consumption. This by extension would suggest that females may have a survival advantage over males due to their greater relative fat stores.Most important factor of all, however, appears to be hydration.

In the example that started this post, Rita Chretien survived her 48 day ordeal in large part due to the availability to some melted snow for drinking. Indeed, had no water been available, Rita may not have fared as well. In examples of hospitalized individuals who are in a persistent vegetative state, who become cut off from artificial sustenance, death ensues within 10-14 days. Keep in mind that these individuals are in a coma and completely immobile, thereby consuming the lowest amount of energy possible. It can thus be surmised that the same conditions (no food or water) in a person who is at least somewhat active, and who may perspire, would only lead to a much swifter end.For individuals who like to get out into the wilderness, and who upon reading accounts of other's misadventures (Into the Wild, 127 Hours, etc.) are not in the least discouraged from following suit (present company included), ensuring to always have a reasonable supply of water should be priority number one. Additionally, as is well documented in the eventual demise of Christopher McCandless (Into the Wild) the avoidance of eating unknown plants and shrubs can also be a key survival strategy.

CHAPTER 3

THE SCIENCE STUDY

39) Why its difficult to "burn off" belly fat,and how cell behaved :

Weight is obviously connected to belly fat a we know today.But in early 2016, scientists debunked body-mass index (BMI), a calculation of someone's percentage of body fat based on their height and weight, as a measure (paywall) of overall health. The authors argued that having a high BMI didn't necessarily mean that patients faced the same health risks that obesity can lead to; conversely, having a low BMI didn't mean that patients were healthier.We all need some fat. It's an important component of cell membranes, a place to store energy and some vitamins, and it's used to make different hormones we need to transmit messages throughout the body.Yet higher percentages of body fat above 25% for men and 30% for women can be a health hazard. This is especially the case if it's stored in our upper bodies or around our internal organs, which can cause myriad problems ranging from increased risk of diabetes, heart disease, and cancer.If you want to shed fat, it's important to understand just how the fat cells in our bodies work.

a) Number of fat cell stays the same after weight loss-

In 2008, Kirsty Spalding, a molecular biologist studying fat at the Karolinska Institute in Sweden, made a fascinating discovery: No matter whether we gain or lose weight over time,as an adult ,we maintained same number of fat cells.Spalding observed that from infant to early 20s, the number of fat cells in our bodies increase.But once we reach our mid-20s, though, we keep the same number of fat cells. Though some cells may die, our bodies will replace them quickly. "It's like we are programmed to have the same number of fat cells," she said. Scientists are not sure why some people have more fat cells than others. (They are also not sure if our bodies replace fat cells after undergoing liposuction.)

These fat cells alone aren't a bad thing. When fat becomes a part of our bodies, it's called adipose tissue. Stephen Neabore, a physician at Barnard Medical Center, said that this tissue is comparable to an organ because of all the jobs it carries out.

Over half of our brains are made of fat cells, and fat cells support in our nerve development and function. We also need fat to develop hormones, which serve as the body's chemical signals between different types of tissues. It provides cushioning for our internal organs, almost like shock absorbers, while we do things like run or jump. Also, some kinds of fat can act as insulation from the cold, especially in infants.

Fat cell is also a efficient way to store a lot of energy in a micro space. Chemically, the fat we eat (usually in the form of fatty acids) are chains of hydrogen and carbon attached to a sugar-alcohol molecule. The energy we get from fat—usually around nine calories per gram—comes from the way that our bodies break down the bonds that hold the chains together. Other sources of food, like carbohydrates and proteins, only contain about four calories per gram. Neabore explained that fat around our belly, thighs, and buttocks is a healthy reserve of energy in many case.

To a certain extent, our weight is related to both the number and the size of our fat cells: When we put on weight, we store the extra lipids we don't use in our fat cells, which make them grow in size. As we lose it, fat cells shrink, but will never disappear. This means that two people with similar body shapes could have drastically different numbers of fat cells, depending on how many lipids are stored in those cells.

As a result of Spalding's discovery, this indicated that it may be difficult to keep weight off once we've lost it. "If you can't get rid of these cells, you're just going to have these cells sitting there, constantly saying they want to be bigger," she said.

Spalding said that one of the hormones that fat cells produce is known as leptin, which indicate to our brains that we should stop eating. As they shrink, they produce less of this hormone, which means we may be inclined to eat more, growing the fat cells to their "happy size," as Spalding put it. The best thing to do is to make sure kids maintain a healthy weight, since those who overweight are more likely (paywall) to be overweight as adults.

b)The right foods to strike a balance-

Our primary resting energy source is a chemical called glycogen, which is a chain of sugars our bodies can make from food. One of the many jobs of our liver is to store glycogen for later use. Neabore said, "During the day when we eat, most of the simple sugars—or complex sugars, either way—work to refill our glycogen stores...When your liver is all the way full, the rest of what you're trying to contribute will eventually get turned into fat."

When we engage in an activity that requires energy, our bodies to use chemicals from the food we eat. It's easiest to break down carbohydrates, but once we've gone through all the energy we can get from carbs (after roughly 20 to 45 minutes of exercise), our bodies move on to consuming fat, in the form of extra lipids, from our adipose tissue. Burning these lipids is what causes us to lose weight—assuming we don't consume more to replace it. Weight loss is attributed to fat cells shrinking, not losing them entirely.

For the general population trying to maintain a healthy weight, (excluding those suffering from eating disorders or malnutrition) Neabore recommends a plant-based diet. This includes grains, fruits, vegetables, nuts, seeds, and beans.

"Fat is one of the basic building blocks of food, and all naturally occurring foods are made of some combination of [fat, carbohydrates, and protein]," he said. We're able to get all of the nutrients we need from plants. Neabore says that if you're trying to lose fat, it's a good idea to avoid foods that are high in fat, which tend to include animal products, like beef. Though foods like meat and fish can also be nutritious, "you want to let your body burn off the fat it already has, and you don't want to add more to your stockpile."

40) Thin people may be fat on the inside, doctors warn :

If it really is what's on the inside that counts, then a lot of thin people might be in trouble.Some doctors now believe the internal fat surrounding vital organs like the heart, liver or pancreas— invisible to the naked eye— could be as dangerous as the more obvious external fat that bulges underneath the skin."Being thin doesn't automatically mean you're not fat," said Dr. Jimmy Bell, a professor of molecular imaging at Imperial College, London.Since 1994, Bell and his team have scanned nearly 800 people with MRI machines to create "fat maps" showing where people store fat.According to the data, people who maintain their weight through diet rather than exercise are likely to have major deposits of internal fat, even if they are otherwise slim.

"The whole concept of being fat needs to be redefined," said Bell, whose research is funded by Britain's Medical Research Council.Without a clear warning signallike a rounder middle,doctors worry that thin people may be lulled into falsely assuming that because they're not overweight, they're healthy."Just because someone is lean doesn't make them immune to diabetes or other risk factors for heart disease," said Dr. Louis Teichholz, chief of cardiology at Hackensack University Medical Center in New Jersey, who was not involved in Bell's research.

a) Internal fat found in models-

Even people with normal Body Mass Index scores— a standard obesity measure that divides your weight by the square of your height— can have surprising levels of fat deposits inside.Of the women scanned by Bell and his colleagues, as many as 45 per cent of those with normal BMI scores (20 to 25) actually had excessive levels of internal fat. Among men, the percentage was nearly 60 per cent.Relating the news to what Bell calls TOFIs— people who are "thin outside, fat inside"— is rarely uneventful.

"The thinner people are, the bigger the surprise," he said, adding the researchers even found TOFIs among people who are professional models.According to Bell, people who are fat on the inside are essentially on the threshold of being obese. They eat too many fatty, sugary foods— and exercise too little to work it off— but they are not eating enough to actually be fat.Scientists believe we naturally accumulate fat around the belly first, but at some point, the body may start storing it elsewhere.Still, most experts believe that being of normal weight is an indicator of good health, and that BMI is a reliable measurement.

"BMI won't give you the exact indication of where fat is, but it's a useful clinical tool," said Dr. Toni Steer, a nutritionist at Britain's Medical Research Council.

b) Mistaken signals for fat storage-

Doctors are unsure about the exact dangers of internal fat, but some suspect it contributes to the risk of heart disease and diabetes.They theorize that internal fat disrupts the body's communication systems. The fat enveloping internal organs might be sending the body mistaken chemical signals to store fat inside organs like the liver or pancreas. This could ultimately lead to insulin resistance, Type 2 diabetes or heart disease.Experts have long known that fat, active people can be healthier than their skinny, inactive counterparts.

"Normal-weight persons who are sedentary and unfit are at much higher risk for mortality than obese persons who are active and fit," said Dr. Steven Blair, an obesity expert at the University of South Carolina.The good news is that internal fat can be easily burned off through exercise or even by improving your diet."Even if you don't see it on your bathroom scale, caloric restriction and physical exercise have an aggressive effect on visceral fat," said Dr. Bob Ross, an obesity expert at Queen's University in Kingston, Ont.Because many factors contribute to heart disease, Teichholz says it's difficult to determine the precise danger of internal fat, though it certainly doesn't help."Obesity is a risk factor, but it's lower down on the totem pole of risk factors," he said.

He explained that whether people smoke, their family histories, and blood pressure and cholesterol rates are more important determinants than both external and internal fat.

41) Scientists discover why thin people dislike fat people:

From playground taunts to discrimination at work, prejudice is a fact of life for millions who are overweight.Now scientists claim to have discovered why.While it will be of little comfort to anyone who has been bullied over their weight, it is suggested that thinner humans have an inbuilt dislike of fat people because of ancient fears that they may be diseased.Researchers found that the mere sight of someone who is overweight can trigger feelings of disgust and nausea similar to encountering rotten food.The research, reported in the journal Evolution and Human Behaviour, claims that our brains have evolved to react to outward signs of disease, such as rashes and wounds, because bacteria and viruses are invisible.

Unfortunately, these signals also include excessive body fat."Antipathy towards obese people is a powerful and pervasive prejudice in many contemporary populations," said the team from the University of British Columbia."Our results reveal, for the first time, that this prejudice may be rooted in multiple, independent mechanisms."A questionnaire found that feelings of disgust towards the obese were strongest in people with the greatest fear of disease.Those who agreed with comments such as "it really bothers me when people sneeze without covering their mouths" were more likely to agree with statements such as "if I were an employer looking to hire, I might avoid hiring a fat person".

Last night, TV presenter-Anne Diamond, who helps people conquer obesity after briefly ballooning to 14st 9lb herself, said: "The research sounds reasonable enough I suppose; obesity is unhealthy and if there is something in us that helps us avoid ill health I can understand that."But I don't believe that in the 21st century we can use it as an excuse for prejudice."Obesity is an illness, but something becoming so common that it will soon be the norm."

42) Fat people are actually nicer than thin people, according to science:

If you're carrying a few extra pounds, you're much more likely to be generous with pounds sterling, a new study suggests. Thin people are basically stingy, miserable gits. German researchers asked 20 fat men (weighing in at an average of 19 stone) and 20 thin men (weighing in at an average of 11) to play lab games where they offered people money. The researchers found that, 'lean men made less fair decisions and offered 16 per cent less money than corpulent men' In particular, thin people tended to give more money to other thin people – and tended to be more grumpy when they had low blood sugar levels. MORE: Vegans are like a 'sect' and should all be killed, top chef says The researchers write: 'Our data show that economic decision-making is affected by both the body weight of the participants and the body weight of their opponents, and that blood glucose concentrations should be taken into consideration when analysing economic decision making.'

43) Characteristics of metabolically unhealthy lean people

Compared to people who are of normal weight and metabolically healthy, subjects who are of normal weight but metabolically unhealthy (~20% of normal weight adults) have a more than three-fold higher risk of mortality and/or cardiovascular events. This risk is also higher than that of metabolically healthy obese subjects. Norbert Stefan, Fritz Schick and Hans-Ulrich Häring have now addressed characteristics determining metabolic health in lean, overweight and obese people, showed that a reduced accumulation of fat in the lower body puts lean people at risk and highlighted implications of their findings for personalized prevention and treatment of cardiometabolic diseases.

It has now been established that a body-mass index (BMI) in the normal weight range (defined by WHO as a BMI of $18 \cdot 5 - < 25 \cdot 0$ kg/m^2) associates with the lowest all-cause mortality. However, does this assumption apply to all subjects in this BMI range? The research into the causes and consequences of metabolically healthy obesity (MHO) has shown that for a certain BMI, the risk of cardiometablic disease and death can vary substantially among subjects. In this respect, large studies showed that, compared to metabolically healthy people in the normal weight range, subjects with MHO only have a moderate (~25%) higher risk of all-cause mortality and/or cardiovascular events, while the risk is much higher (~300%) in metabolically unhealthy lean people. This raises four important question: 1. what phenotypes characterize these metabolically unhealthy lean people, 2. do these phenotypes differ from those which place obese subjects at increased risk, 3. what molecular mechanisms determine these phenotypes in lean and in obese subjects and 4. how can this knowledge be used to prevent and treat diseases?

The researchers from the Department of Internal Medicine IV of the University Hospital Tübingen and the Institute for Diabetes Research and Metabolic Diseases (IDM) of the Helmholtz Centre Munich, a partner of the German Center for Diabetes Research (DZD), have now analyzed data from 981 subjects. After having defined metabolic health as having less than 2 risk parameters of the metabolic syndrome, they found that 18% of their lean subjects were metabolically unhealthy. This number perfectly matches the numbers detected in larger studies that investigated the relationship of metabolic health with cardiovascular events and mortality.

Stefan and colleagues now used magnetic resonance imaging and magnetic resonance spectroscopy to precisely determine body fat mass, fat distribution and deposition of fat in the liver. Furthermore, they determined insulin sensitivity, insulin secretion, thickness of the carotid vessel wall and fitness. They found that among the fat compartments a low percentage leg fat mass was the strongest determinant of metabolic risk in lean subjects, while in obese subjects nonalcoholic fatty liver disease and increased intra-abdominal fat mass strongly determined this risk. Based on these findings, and with support from animal data and genetic data from human studies, they concluded that in lean subjects the problem of storing fat in the leg may be a crucial factor placing lean people at increased risk of cardiometabolic diseases. They further hypothesize that this phenotype resembles the phenotypes observed in some very rare diseases, called lipodystrophy. However, they highlight that this lipodystrophy-like phenotype has a much less severe form that the ones observed in these diseases.

In respect to the impact of their findings for routine clinical practice the researchers make the following points: First, in the case that a subject with normal weight may have two or more parameters of the metabolic syndrome in a clinical examination, and/or may have a low leg fat mass, it would be important to perform careful diagnostics to early detect metabolic diseases. Second, if a cardiometabolic disease, such as type 2 diabetes or cardiovascular disease, is present in very lean people, pharmacological treatment resulting in an increase in subcutaneous fat mass may be beneficial for some patients. In this respect thiazolidinediones may be of major interest. Finally, applying well-defined phenotyping strategies in clinical trials to better separate the metabolic risk in lean and obese subjects may help to better tailor lifestyle and pharmacological intervention to accomplish the goal of providing personalized prevention and treatment to the patients.

44) Fat? Thin? Molecular switch may turn obesity on or off:

Identical twins may be alike in everything from their eye color to their favorite foods, but they can diverge in one important characteristic: their weight. A new study uncovers a molecular mechanism for obesity that might explain why one twin can be extremely overweight even while the other is thin.Heredity influences whether we become obese, but the genes researchers have linked to the condition don't explain many of the differences in weight among people. Identical twins with nonidentical weights are a prime example. So what accounts for the variation? Changes in the intestinal microbiome—the collection of bacteria living in the gut—are one possibility. Another is epigenetic changes, or alterations in gene activity. These changes occur when molecules latch on to DNA or the proteins it wraps around, turning sets of genes "on" or "off."

Triggered by factors in the environment, epigenetic modifications can be passed down from one generation to the next. This type of transmission happened during the Hunger Winter, a famine that occurred when the Germans cut off food supplies to parts of the Netherlands in the final months of World War II. Mothers who were pregnant during the famine gave birth to children who were prone to obesity decades later, suggesting that the mothers' diets had a lasting impact on their kids' metabolism. However, which epigenetic changes in people promote obesity remains unclear.So when—many decades later—physiologist J. Andrew Pospisilik of the Max Planck Institute of Immunobiology and Epigenetics in Freiburg, Germany, and colleagues noticed an odd pattern of weight gain in some mutant mice, they were intrigued. The mice had only one copy of a gene called Trim28, and the researchers found that most them were either obese or lean, with few animals in between.

To discover why, the scientists measured gene activity in the animals. Trim28 controls the activity of several other genes, making it an epigenetic modifier. In the obese mice, the activity of an interacting set of genes was turned down. Previous studies have implicated these genes in body weight management, and some are activated in fat cells and the hypothalamus, the brain area that triggers hunger. The functions of the genes remain unclear, but Pospisilik and colleagues hypothesize that Trim28 helps form an epigenetic switch that can flip on obesity by suppressing these genes.But could the same mechanism foster obesity in humans? After all, the mice have only one copy of the Trim28 gene, whereas people have two copies. To find out, the team took fat samples from children who were in the hospital for surgery. TRIM28 activity was abnormally low in fat from kids who were obese. "There's a subset of children who look very much like the obese mice" in their TRIM28 measurements, Pospisilik says. The researchers also analyzed data on 13 pairs of identical twins in which one twin was obese. TRIM28 activity was diminished in fat from the obese twins, the scientists report online today in Cell.

"We show that you can have a strong phenotype [obesity] with absolutely no genetic underpinnings," Pospisilik says. He notes that researchers used to think that epigenetic effects might tweak our weight by only a few kilograms. But if people gained an amount of weight equivalent to what the mice gained, he says, it would mean the difference between being "on the rugby team instead of the badminton team." "The study gives us a new potential mechanism of obesity," says genetic epidemiologist Jeanne McCaffery of Brown University who wasn't connected to the research. And that could be good news for researchers who are looking for ways to prevent or reverse the condition, she says. "There may be multiple subtypes of obesity that may be amenable to different treatments." Pospisilik suggests several risk factors for obesity in children, such as their mothers' smoking and eating habits during pregnancy. But "the big question now is what is the trigger" that flips the obesity switch, says genetic epidemiologist Paul Franks of the Lund University Diabetes Center in Malmö, Sweden. "If you could determine what that was, you'd have the basis for intervention."

45) To Lose and Keep Off Weight, Turn Off Your Body's 'Fat Switch':

Most people don't think about fat insects or hibernating animals when they talk about the cause of obesity, so it's refreshing to see a book that tackles obesity as a normal process that all animals have learned.In his new book The Fat Switch, Richard J. Johnson, a professor of medicine and head of the division of Renal Diseases and Hypertension at the University of Colorado-Denver, argues that obesity is a process animals have used to protect themselves during periods of food shortage, and that they have learned to "flip" a switch when they want to gain weight. The switch occurs in the energy factories of the body (mitochondria) and results in the desire to eat more than is needed and to reduce energy output, thus allowing the maximal conversion of food into fat.

The usual argument is that people gain weight because they eat too much and exercise too little. They blame large portions of food, supersize drinks, TV, the Internet and video games. But Johnson says the real reason people are getting fat is that they have inadvertently activated the "fat switch." In other words, we are eating more not because we are given bigger servings of food, but because we demand bigger servings, and we are exercising less not because we are watching more TV, but we are watching more TV because we have less energy.So what flips the fat switch? In a word: sugar. More precisely, says Johnson, it is the excessive uric acid that results from excessive sugar consumption. For years, we have heard messages about watching our saturated fat intake. But in reality, sugar is the real cause of our expanding waistlines.

"Fat is the fuel, but sugar, and in particular, fructose, is the fire," says Johnson. "Foods rich in fructose can activate the fat switch — resulting in loss of appetite control and a reduction in energy."The major sources of fructose are table sugar (sucrose, which contains glucose and fructose), and cheap, ubiquitous high-fructose corn syrup (HFCS), which is often added to foods to enhance taste. Fructose can also be generated from carbohydrate-heavy diets. "In the big picture," said Johnson in an interview, "it's sugar and high-fructose corn syrup driving this obesity epidemic. But you can make sugar from carbohydrates."Although sugar is the major culprit, Johnson also argues that humans are particularly sensitive to the effects of sugar. He says that millions of years ago, our ancestors dwelled in rainforests and subsisted on fructose from natural fruits. But global cooling led to disappearing rainforests and famine during the colder months when fruits were unavailable. This led to a genetic mutation that resulted in a greater uric acid response to fructose. "This mutation was life-saving," Johnson explained, "as it allowed animals to convert fat much more effectively from fruit."All was well for millions of years — until the discovery of sugar cane and, with it, plentiful fructose. Today, one can drink huge amounts in one supergulp soft drink. And we have become super-effective at converting the fructose to fat. "So what was life-saving in the past," says Johnson, "is driving obesity today — a great irony."

Making matters worse, the more sugar we eat, the more uric acid our bodies produce, which increases our liver and intestines' ability to absorb sugar. "Obese people absorb fructose more easily," says Johnson, "whereas skinny people don't absorb it very well."If nothing changes, Johnson told me, it becomes "like a snowball rolling down the hill." He explained, "The more sugar you eat, the more uric acid you make. And the more uric acid, the more metabolism of fructose that occurs."Once the snowball has increased in size and speed, it's harder to stop it. "In the early phase of obesity," says Johnson, "if you cut out the foods you recover your weight. But over time, it looks like you lose [the energy-producing mitochondria] and can't recover them. It seems you reset yourself to a higher weight."The net effect: an increase in fat accumulation, insulin resistance (Type 2 diabetes), higher blood pressure and triglycerides, and stimulation of low-grade inflammation that activates the immune system. Coronary artery disease, strokes, aortic aneurysms and congestive heart failure are just some of the complications linked to sugar-fueled obesity.If this all seems bleak and hopeless, take heart. Johnson suggests in The Fat Switch that keeping the switch off — which is essential for good health — depends on following a few general principles.

Of course, reducing your intake of added sugars is key. Johnson recommends no more than four to five teaspoons per day. "The first step is to eliminate soft drinks and fruit punches with added sugars," he writes, "as the effects of fructose relate to the concentration that the liver is exposed to, and this relates not only to the amount ingested but also the rate. However, natural fruits are OK as they have a lot of good ingredients like vitamin C and antioxidants that block the effects of sugar."Another important step is to reduce carbohydrates — but only at certain times of the day. "I think most people would like to maintain a normal balance of only 25 to 30 percent carbohydrates, at least 15 percent protein and the rest fat," says Johnson. "However, the key way to lose weight is to simply restrict the carbohydrates for two of the three meals of the day. This allows the body to burn fat for much of the day." At least 30 minutes of exercise and at least eight hours of sleep every day have additional health benefits.

Johnson recommends limiting purine-rich beer because it increases uric acid production. Interestingly, both regular beer and nonalcoholic beer are problems, because the purines are from the brewer's yeast, not from the alcohol. Do, however, drink milk and eat cheese, as they are associated with reduced risk for obesity, diabetes and gout. Coffee drinking also appears to reduce the risk of developing diabetes, and is likewise associated with lower uric acid levels.Eating a quarter of a big bar of 70 percent dark chocolate per day appears to replenish the cell mitochondria needed to control fat production. In fact Johnson says research is showing that the flavinol in dark chocolate, epicatechin, can actually block many of the effects of fructose — in studies of rats, so far. Even more promising, he writes, "Epicatechin appears to be one of the most potent stimuli to grow mitochondria that has ever been discovered. It may improve muscle mass and exercise performance of aging mice. And it has been shown to increase mitochondrial function in human patients with heart failure."With promising discoveries like these, Johnson told me, "It's really an exciting time." Most exciting of all, as he writes in The Fat Switch, "For those of you who wish to see the day when obesity can be cured, I believe it will not be long."

The Fat Switch is available in hardcover at Mercola.com and Kindle e-book at Amazon.com.

46) Is a Slim Physique Contagious?:

What makes some people slender and others full-figured? Besides diet and genetics, the community of microbes that lives inside us may be partially responsible. New research on twins suggests that lean people harbor bacteria that their obese counterparts don't have. And, given the chance, those bacteria may be able to prevent weight gain. But don't dig your skinny jeans out of the closet just yet. So far, the work has been done only in mice. What's more, the bacterial takeover requires a healthy, high-fiber diet to work, illustrating the complex relationship between diet, microbes, metabolism, and health.Our intestines are home to at least 400 species of bacteria, and evidence is building that the balance of microbes in our internal ecosystem has far-reaching effects on health, including brain function and risk of cancer. A study last year showed that transferring gut bacteria between humans reduced insulin resistance, which is linked to obesity.

To explore how microbes differ between obese and lean people, researchers at Washington University in St. Louis took gut bacteria from four pairs of identical and fraternal twins; one sibling in each pair was lean and the other obese. Then they transplanted these microbes into mice that had no intestinal microbes of their own. The mice who got microbes from the lean twins stayed lean, the researchers report today in Science. Those that got microbes from the obese twins increased their body fat by 10% on average, even though they were eating the same amount of food.What would happen if these two sets of microbes got mixed up in the gut, the researchers wondered. Led by microbiologist Jeffrey Gordon and graduate student Vanessa Ridaura, the team took advantage of one of the rodents' least endearing habits: They eat each other's poop. After letting this happen, the researchers discovered that microbes from the lean twins seemed to be particularly good at taking hold in the gut ecosystems of the mice that started with obesity-associated microbes. And after those bacteria moved in, the mice didn't gain weight. The most invasive species of microbes from the thin animals were in the Bacteroidetes group, which has previously been associated with leanness in mice and humans. The obese mice seemed to have unoccupied niches that the Bacteroidetes could easily move into.

To figure out what the gut bacteria might be doing, the researchers looked for bacterial genes that were active in the two kinds of mice. The heavier mice had higher levels of proteins involved in detoxification and stress responses; the lean mice expressed more genes involved in breaking down dietary fiber.Diet, it turns out, was key to the impressive properties of the microbes from the lean twins. All the mice in the first round of experiments had been eating chow that was high in fiber and low in fat. The researchers then prepared a mouse-pellet form of an unhealthy human diet, high in fat and low in fiber, and housed svelte and heavy mice together again. They found that, with this diet, the microbes associated with leanness didn't colonize the cagemates' intestines.

This work was rigorously done and fits in well with earlier findings, including the idea that Bacteroides may protect against weight gain, says Alan Walker, a gut microbiologist at the Wellcome Trust Sanger Institute in the United Kingdom who was not involved in the study. What's new here, he says, is that the researchers began addressing the question of how that protection might work: which species are responsible, what genes they use, and what diet they require."This study is an important step toward ultimately answering these questions," says microbiologist Peter Turnbaugh of Harvard University. A valuable result of this work, they both agree, is that it sets up a way to test the effects of microbial therapies on human gut bacteria (even though the bugs are living in a mouse). The authors suggest that a logical next step is to use the animals to measure the effects of particular foods or ingredients on gut ecosystems.

The mouse experiments also provide a way to test fecal transplants, which can cure a potentially fatal intestinal infection in humans and show potential for treating other conditions such as inflammatory bowel disease and obesity. There's a danger inherent in this approach: Transferring human feces into a patient's colon runs the risk of transmitting pathogens as well. Walker and the authors note that a well-tested "next-generation probiotic" consisting of known beneficial microbes delivered as a pill or other therapy could take the place of fresh feces, and this mouse system provides a way to identify the most effective bacteria, the diseases those bacteria can treat, and whether a particular diet is necessary.

There's a major way to go before you can translate these results to humans," Walker cautions. A weight-loss probiotic isn't a simple next step, as the researchers found when they isolated 39 of the beneficial Bacteroidetes species. The mixture was unable to cause the same effects as mouse poop, possibly because the Bacteroidetes aren't acting alone and more of the microbial players need to be identified.

47) Obesity researchers study thin people for clues about hunger and metabolism:

Maureen Michael likes food. Most days, she has three or four meals, and on occasion she eats yet another in the middle of the night. But she rarely worries about her weight, and at 5-foot-8 and 155 pounds, she looks quite trim."I eat anything, and I eat a lot," the 51-year-old District resident said. "I like large portions. I have one of those metabolisms, I guess."Just the other day, Michael ate a salad and two large helpings of spaghetti and meatballs for dinner — after having a hearty bowl of ice cream. For breakfast the next morning, she ate two scrambled eggs, half a package of Polish sausage, English muffins and orange juice. For lunch, she consumed a 12-inch seafood sub and some Doritos, and that night's dinner featured two pork chops, potatoes and broccoli.

That Michael's weight remains steady even though she eats whatever she wants and does not exercise interests scientists studying the nation's obesity epidemic. By looking at people who are near their ideal body weight, these researchers at the National Institutes of Health's Metabolic Clinical Research Unit in Bethesda hope to figure out what causes so many others to be overweight or uncontrollably fat.Michael is among the one-third of American adults who are at a good weight relative to their height and build. Another third are overweight, and the rest are obese. Unlike Michael, very few people keep their weight in check without paying attention to what they eat and being conscientious about physical activity.

For years, people have been told to diet, control their appetites, use a little willpower. But more and more scientists believe the obesity epidemic has been triggered by a combination beyond an individual's control: genes, and how they interact with an environment of abundant, tasty, inexpensive and hard-to-resist food.Each person's unique genetic makeup, these experts think, may affect what he craves, how much he craves and how his body uses fat and burns calories."We are hard-wired to be a bit more hungry than we need to, because until very recently — in evolutionary terms — the vast majority of our fellow humans had no idea whether the next meal would be available or not," said Francesco S. Celi, a clinical investigator at the NIH research unit

Yet for some people, there is a profound imbalance between what they eat and the amount of energy they expend. Most of these people become obese as a result, but some, like Michael, don't."Some are more sensitive" to that imbalance, said Rudolph Leibel, a diabetes researcher at New York's Columbia University who has been studying the biochemistry and genetics of obesity for 25 years. "That's the genetics.""There are people in the population who are skinnier or more slender with a different genetic response to the environment," he said. That is why "just yelling at people and telling them it is sinful or gluttony is not a particular fruitful way to deal with the problem. It's not very effective to insinuate that someone has moral failings when a behavior is involved."

To try to unravel the complexity of all this, researchers at an NIH diabetes and obesity lab in Phoenix have begun to incorporate thin people into their studies. Why "some [people] tend to overeat more than they need more consistently and why this occurs is clearly complex and involves levels of behavior that we are just beginning to understand," said Jonathan Krakoff, an endocrinologist at the lab.Krakoff and his colleagues are recruiting for a study in which thin people will consume about 4,000 calories in a 24-hour period, about twice the amount an average healthy person needs in a day.Before participants engage in the overeating part of the study, researchers will measure their body fat and will conduct a test to make sure they don't have diabetes or impaired glucose tolerance. Then, scientists will count how many calories the participants burn in a day while they're studied. This measurement is done in a respiratory chamber where the amount of oxygen taken in and carbon dioxide expelled is monitored, revealing the number of calories burned.

"Some people might be able to burn off more excess calories as heat when they overeat, so they are the people more likely to be thin," said Marie Thearle, a staff clinician involved in the study. "We are also asking our volunteers to come back for follow-up visits once a year for up to seven years to see if any of the energy expenditure measurements with overeating during the baseline study visit predict who gains weight over time and who does not."Thearle hopes to look deeper still into how different bodies use different nutrients, such as carbohydrates, fat and protein, and if food choices matter. "We measure whether the participant's body prefers to use carbohydrates or fat for fuel, and then we further break this down to see how many calories are being used from carbohydrates, fat and protein, respectively."

Thearle says the researchers hope to find out whether food choices matter. "Once you have met the needs of your body, does it matter what else you consume?" she said. "There's the popular myth that people don't gain weight because they have a high metabolism; we want to see if that is true. We will be looking at hormones and brown fat. We don't think the answer is differences in metabolism." Brown fat is the "good" fat that scientists say helps burn calories and white fat, or what we think of as regular fat.A second study at the Phoenix lab, which will involve both slim and obese participants, is more long-range. During a six-week period, the thin people will be fed meals containing 150 percent of their weight-maintaining needs. Some will get a normal amount of protein; for others, the diet will be very low in protein. Obese people will be underfed by "50 percent of their weight-maintaining needs," said Susanne Votruba, a research nutritionist at the lab.

Researchers will analyze every bit of what comes in and out of these participants. "For the long-term study, we measure output (urine and stool) and input (food) . . . to determine the exact calories that are going in and out," Vortuba wrote in an e-mail.Vortuba hopes to figure out who among the thin volunteers gains more weight over time, and why, and who among the fatter volunteers loses more weight, and why.

In Bethesda, Celi and another investigator, Kong Chen, are taking a slightly different approach. Since humans spend so much time at rest and since "obesity is an imbalance between energy intake and energy expenditure," Celi said, he and Chen are testing what happens to a person's output of energy, stress hormones and thyroid hormone levels when his or her body gets cold.Some studies suggest that colder temperatures help stimulate brown fat to burn more calories. Brown fat, which runs along our neck, shoulders and spine in small amounts, is like muscle tissue in that it burns calories and helps keep the body's internal temperature stable. Only recently have scientists discovered that brown fat persists in humans beyond infancy.They have also found that lean people tend to have more brown fat than obese people.

If temperatures can influence brown fat so that the body expends more energy, people with a lot of brown fat may find it easier to lose or maintain their weight, Celi and Chen believe. If that is the case, then "instead of working on hunger, which is deep-seated in the brain," Celi said, "we are working on one tissue [brown fat] that has been proposed as the holy grail of the [human metabolic] system. We bypass the brain."Michael is one of 24 lean recruits in a preliminary experiment run by Celi and Chen. She spent two 12-hour overnights in a specialized room with precise temperature and airflow controls. During each session inside the chamber, she ate a diet of 55 percent carbohydrates, 35 percent fat and 15 to 20 percent protein — just enough, the scientists calculated, for her to maintain her weight — while they held the room temperature at 75 degrees for one session and 68 degrees for the other.All the while, they measured her oxygen and carbon dioxide output. They calculated her body mass. She spent 10 minutes in an oval-shape, space-age-looking machine called a Bod-Pod, which computed the weight and volume of her fat composition. She swallowed a pill containing a sensor that traced her internal temperature, while patches placed on her skin gauged her external temperature. Her heart was constantly assessed, and every 30 minutes small amounts of fluids were collected from fat tissue around her belly to evaluate her metabolism. Blood and urine samples were also taken.

Another participant, Chris Nathasingh — 31 years old, 5-11 and 170 pounds — spent his 68-degree night with only a thin blanket to supplement his pajamas. He shivered and jumped in and out of bed to keep warmThe next morning, he was exhausted but not very hungry. The second night, the temperature was adjusted to 75 degrees, and Nathasingh slept well. "I would not say that I was hungry or hungrier [after the second night], but I definitely could not wait to eat," he said. "Where sleep deprivation after the cold night made me only focus on sleep, the absence of such deprivation after the warm night made me focus on the next best thing: food."Celi and Chen are optimistic about some early findings in the trial. The participants' energy expenditures went up when the room temperature was lowered. They plan to conduct a larger study, involving 180 volunteers, both lean and overweight.

Michael, who was a swimmer, dancer and gymnast as a girl, and who was skinnier than her girlhood friends, keeps her home at about 72 degrees in the winter (a bit warmer than she likes, but her elderly mother likes it warm) and about 70 degrees in the summer. Her weight is a little higher than she wants, but she doesn't think about dieting. Instead, she might try some exercise.

"I need to," she said. "I am getting older. I have slacked off as an adult. I can tell the difference."

48) Why Thin Will Always Be In:

A recent study published in the Archives of Internal Medicine reported that not all overweight people are necessarily at higher risk for cardiovascular diseases. This is being translated into headlines like, "Fit and Fat: Study Shows It's Possible."Of course it's possible; doctors have known for many years that not everyone who is overweight is unhealthy. A person's overall fitness is more important to his or her health than numbers on the scale. For example, most professional football players would be considered overweight, yet they are healthier than average because of their level of fitness.But the problem is that most Americans aren't like professional football players.

Most Americans — fat or thin — are not eating healthy diets, nor are they getting enough exercise. Physically active people are both fitter and thinner than people who do not exercise regularly. Researchers caution that the recent study does not show that being overweight is healthy; in fact, fat people had twice the heart risk as thin people.

Is big beautiful?

There's also of course a social element to obesity. As a nation we keep getting fatter, and for some people that's not a bad thing. Fat-acceptance groups and activists have tried for years to encourage the idea that fat is sexy. Countless books with titles like "Fat Chicks Rule!" and "Embracing Your Fat Ass" promote the message that big is beautiful. While their empowerment message is mixed (it's good to have a positive self-image, but accepting your extra weight may take years off your life), the truth is that the effort has failed.While there is anti-fat bias in the media, anti-thin bias exists as well: Celebrities such as Angelina Jolie, the Olsen twins, and Lindsay Lohan have been regularly mocked and criticized for their thinness. On late night talk shows you are far more likely to hear a joke about how thin Nicole Richie is than a fat joke about how heavy Queen Latifah is.

Ideals of beauty change somewhat over time, but the simple fact is that proponents of plus-size preference have failed to convince America that fat is beautiful. They have tried for years to make fat as sexy as thin. It's no secret that thin people are considered more attractive than fat people.But thin will always be in, for a few simple reasons.

a) Supply and demand-

The first is simple supply and demand. This is pretty easy to grasp — things that are rare (whether diamonds, Picassos, or people with extraordinary sports ability) tend to be more highly valued than things that are common. In our culture (and in many others around the world), the vast majority of people are overweight or obese. Because the average person is overweight, thinner people are by definition rarer, and therefore more in demand. And the fatter our country gets, the more valued thin people will be, based on body shape alone. This isn't a value judgment of worth, it's basic economics.

b) There's also an evolutionary perspective-

At one point in our evolution, people who were heavier than average were prized as mates, clearly having access to food and resources. That is no longer true, and today obesity is instead a strong predictor of health problems; the person of normal weight is, on average, healthier than his or her overweight counterpart. All animals, including humans, choose partners partly (if subconsciously) on reproductive fitness: will this person be healthy enough to carry on my genes?

Note that this bias also works against very thin people. Men are less attracted to unhealthily thin women for the same reason. Studies done by researcher Devendra Singh show that when men are asked to rate the attractiveness of silhouettes of womens' bodies, they overwhelmingly pick the silhouette corresponding with the healthiest weight for women — not too thin, not too fat.

Of course, body shape is only one factor of many, and most overweight people find happiness and love. Being thin is no guarantee of being happy, attractive, or healthy. But, like it or not, there is — and always will be — an advantage to being thin.

49) Skinny and 119 Pounds,but With the Health ,Hallmarks of Obesity:

A small group of thin patients who develop disorders typically tied to obesity pose a medical mystery and a potential opportunity for scientists.Claire Walker Johnson of Queens was a medical mystery. No matter how much she ate, she never gained weight.And yet Ms. Johnson, with a long narrow face, had the conditions many obese people develop — Type 2 diabetes, high blood pressure, high cholesterol and, most strikingly, a liver buried in fat.She and a very small group of very thin people like her have given scientists surprising clues to one of the most important questions about obesity: Why do fat people often develop serious and sometimes life-threatening medical conditions?The answer has little to do with the fat itself. It's about each person's ability to store it. With that understanding, scientists are now working on drug treatments to protect people from excess unstored fat and spare them from dire medical conditions.The need is clear. One in three Americans and one in four adults worldwide have at least three conditions associated with obesity such as diabetes, high cholesterol and high blood pressure — a combination of disorders that doubles their risk of heart attacks and strokes. In addition, 2 percent to 3 percent of adults in

America, or at least five million people, have a grave accumulation of fat in their livers caused by obesity that can lead to liver failure.The detective work that led to this new scientific understanding of fat began with a small group of scientists curious about a disorder that can be caused by a gene mutation so rare it is estimated to affect just one in 10 million people, including, it turned out, Ms. Johnson.

For much of her life, Ms. Johnson, 55, had no idea anything was amiss. Yes, she was very thin and always ravenous, but in Jamaica, where she was born, many children were skinny, she says, and no one thought much of it. She seemed healthy, and she developed normally through adolescence.After coming to the United States as a college student, she saw a doctor for some bumps on her arms and was stunned to learn that they were cholesterol crystallizing from her blood. Her cholesterol level was sky high.Further exams revealed that she had other problems fat people can develop — a huge fatty liver, ovarian cysts, extraordinarily high levels of triglycerides.Ms. Johnson's doctor was baffled. The usual instructions to patients to lose weight made no sense in this case. "He said, 'I don't think I can help you,'" she recalled.She ended up in the office of an endocrinologist, Dr. Maria New, who also was stumped but determined to find answers. She measured Ms. Johnson: 5 feet 7 inches. She weighed her: 119 pounds.Dr. New spent years asking specialists at every medical conference she attended about Ms. Johnson. One day in 1996, she was giving a lecture at the National Institutes of Health and posed her usual query: Did anyone know what might be wrong with her skinny patient?Dr. Simeon Taylor, who was the chief of the diabetes branch at the National Institute of Diabetes and Digestive and Kidney Diseases, popped up from his chair. He had seen several patients like Ms. Johnson. They have lipodystrophy, he said, a rare genetic disorder that is characterized by an abnormal lack of fatty tissue.

Dr. Taylor and his colleagues had been studying people with the disorder "as a curiosity," he told Dr. New. He was interested in insulin resistance, the cause of Type 2 diabetes, and had assumed it resulted from obesity. But people with lipodystrophy had the most severe insulin resistance he had ever seen, and they were far from obese.He was hoping to start a study with a new drug, a synthetic version of a hormone called leptin, that might help the patients. The study began in 2000 with Ms. Johnson as one of its first participants.Leptin is released by fat cells and travels through the blood to the brain. The more fat on a person's body, the more leptin is released. When fat levels are low, leptin levels in the brain are low, and the brain responds by increasing the person's appetite, prompting the person to eat and gain weight. For someone like Ms. Johnson, who has almost no fat cells to signal the brain, the brain gets almost no leptin. To the brain, it seems as if she is starving. As a result, she receives continuous signals to eat.With leptin treatment, Ms. Johnson's brain was tricked into responding as though she had abundant fat. Her insatiable hunger vanished. Fat disappeared from her liver, her blood glucose became normal, and so did her cholesterol and triglyceride levels.

But why did she and other lipodystrophy patients have these conditions in the first place, and why did they vanish? What was going on?A couple of studies involving mice produced some clues. Dr. Marc Reitman, the chief of the diabetes, endocrinology and obesity branch at the National Institute of Diabetes and Digestive and Kidney Diseases and his colleague, Dr. Charles Vinson, of the National Cancer Institute, genetically engineered mice to have lipodystrophy. The mice, like Ms. Johnson, had almost no fat tissue. And like her, they developed all of the conditions associated with obesity.

What would happen, the researchers asked, if the mice had a bit more fat tissue?

They transplanted fat tissue into the rodents, and two weeks later, the mice had normal levels of glucose, insulin and triglycerides. Their livers and muscles went back to normal, too.If that worked, the scientists wondered, could a limitless amount of fat tissue prevent the syndrome, even if copious amounts of fat were stored in that tissue?Philipp E. Scherer, the director of the Touchstone Diabetes Center at the University of Texas Southwestern Medical Center in Dallas, and his colleagues tested the idea. They engineered mice that could make an almost limitless amount of fat tissue. As a result, there was no end to the amount of fat the animals could store. They were, Dr. Scherer said, "the fattest mice under the sun, the mouse equivalent of an 800-pound human being."

The fat mice were metabolically normal -

Now, with years of research, the picture has become clear. And so has a new view of the role of fat itself in causing the medical problems of obesity.At the heart of all these conditions and what is known as "metabolic syndrome," or having at least three of the conditions associated with obesity, is an inadequate ability to store fat. (Dr. C. Ronald Kahn, the chief academic officer of the Joslin Diabetes Clinic, said two German physicians called the syndrome "metabolic" nearly 40 years ago. Conditions like elevated cholesterol, diabetes and even high blood pressure appear to be linked through disruptions in metabolism, in this case the abnormal storage of calories.)The body turns excess food into fat and tries to store it in fat tissue. If there is not enough fat tissue, the fat is stuffed into other organs, like the liver and the heart, as well as the muscles and the pancreas. There it poisons the body, causing metabolic syndrome.

Fat people develop metabolic disorders because their brain is driving them to eat more food than their bodies can store as fat. Their fat tissue has reached its limit. People with lipodystrophy have so little fat tissue that they, too, cannot store the fat their body makes to store extra calories from the food they eat.This is also why some people find that their metabolic disorders improve with just a small weight loss — they are eating less and their fat tissue can respond properly."People traditionally thought of adipose tissue as this inert storage, this white amorphous blob," said Dr. Sam Virtue of the University of Cambridge. In fact, he said, "it is a very dynamic organ."It also explains why 10 percent to 20 percent of obese people never develop metabolic disorders, Dr. Scherer said. These so-called healthy obese are like his fat mice, with an unusual ability to expand their fat tissue to store calories.Now researchers have moved on to the next phase of the investigation, trying to identify the poison in fat that is causing all these problems and find a way to block it. At least two chemicals seem to be involved.

Dr. Gerald I. Shulman, a Yale professor of medicine and co-director of the Diabetes Research Center there, and an investigator at the Howard Hughes Medical Institute, has focused on diacylglycerol, produced from fatty acids — made from the food a person eats — and deposited in places like the muscles and liver instead of fat tissue. With diacylglycerol, Dr. Shulman found, insulin cannot signal cells. The result is insulin resistance and Type 2 diabetes."Diacylglycerol is the culprit," he says. One sure way to get rid of it in liver and muscle cells is to lose weight — to stop providing the body with more calories than its fat tissue can handle, he notes.That is not so easy. "Every patient I see, I say, 'Let's lose some weight and increase activity.' They all nod their heads. 'That's a great idea.' Maybe one in 100 does it, and even when they are successful, we know how easy it is to gain the weight back."Dr. Shulman is exploring another route, developing benign new variants of a toxic drug that he hopes will be safe and will reduce levels of fat and inflammation in the liver. The drug, dinitrophenol, was once widely used as an over-the counter medication for weight loss, but the Food and Drug Administration took it off the market in 1938 after a few people taking it dropped dead from severely high body temperatures.

He and his colleagues have modified dinitrophenol so, at least in rats, it does not raise body temperature or cause weight loss. But it lowers diacylglycerol levels in the liver and cures Type 2 diabetes and nonalcoholic fatty liver disease, and other metabolic problems associated with obesity.The problem will be developing it for humans. Would people want to be in a clinical trial using a variant of a drug that originally had potentially lethal side effects?

"This is a proof of concept," Dr. Shulman says. "I do think this is a way forward."

Others are focusing on another class of compounds, called ceramides. Dr. Scherer, who is studying them, says they are produced from fat floating in the blood and are unable to get into fat tissue for storage or degradation. They, too, cause insulin resistance. Ceramides can also kill cells if their levels become high and can bring on inflammatory responses. And inflammation, Dr. Scherer adds, is a hallmark of obesity.He and others are looking for the best drugs to stanch the activity of enzymes used to make ceramides. Like Dr. Shulman, he finds that he can show that his idea works in mice. But, he says, "that's easy to do in a mouse."All of this raises a provocative question. "It is so accepted that obesity is bad for you, but why is it bad for you?" Dr. Virtue says. "If I put a 50-pound weight on your back and asked you to walk around all day, you would be a superhealthy person."And that, says Dr. Rudolph Leibel of Columbia University, is the beauty of the work on lipodystrophy. People like Ms. Johnson have shown a pathway that leads to the diseases of obesity.

"The first step toward curing it is to know why," Dr. Leibel says.

50) Diet Myth News Flash: Eating Less Does Not Cause Fat Loss:

I'm all about shattering diet myths.For example, you may have already seen the news flash that snacking doesn't actually increase your metabolism, despite the fact that most "diet experts" tell you to graze on several small meals per day to keep that metabolic fire stoked.Today, I've got another diet myth news flash for you: eating less does not cause fat loss.Yes, you heard me right. You're about to find out why eating less does not cause fat loss – but first you should know that today's diet myth comes straight from Jonathan Bailor, author of a brand new book that I highly recommend you check out: "The Calorie Myth: How To Eat More, Exercise Less, Lose Weight and Live Better.

Why You're Losing Muscle, Not Fat.Let's begin with a quote:

"The reduction of energy intake continues to be the basis of...weight reduction programs...[The results] are known to be poor and not long-lasting."

– George Bray, Pennington Biomedical Research Center

Eating less does not create the need to burn body fat. Instead, it creates the need for the body to slow down. Contrary to popular opinion, the body hangs on to body fat. Instead, it burns muscle tissue, and that worsens the underlying cause of obesity. Only as a last resort, if the body has no other option, it may also burn a bit of body fat. Why does the body hang on to body fat and burn muscle? To answer that question, let's look at it another way. What does our metabolism want more of when it thinks we are starving? Stored energy. What is a great source of stored energy? Body fat. So when our metabolism thinks we are starving, does it want to get rid of or hold on to body fat? It wants to hold on. Next, what does our metabolism want less of when we are starving? It wants less tissue (which burns a lot of calories). What type of tissue burns a lot of calories? Muscle tissue. So when our metabolism thinks we are starving, it gets rid of calorie-hungry muscle tissue. Studies show that up to 70% of the weight lost while eating less comes from burning muscle—not body fat!

Burning all this muscle means that starving ourselves leads to more body fat—not less—over the long term. As soon as we stop starving ourselves, we have all the calories we used to have but need less of them, thanks to all that missing muscle and our slowed-down metabolism. Now our metabolism sees eating a normal amount as overeating and creates new body fat. In the Journal of the American Medical Association, researcher G.L. Thorpe tells us that eating less does not make us lose weight, "...by selective reduction of adipose deposits [body fat], but by wasting of all body tissues...therefore, any success obtained must be maintained by chronic under-nourishment." It is not practical or healthy to keep ourselves "chronically under-nourished," so we don't. Instead, we yo-yo diet. And that is why eating less is not an effective long-term fat loss approach.

The Bad Side Effects Of Food Deprivation -

Imagine watching TV and seeing a commercial for a new medication. The ad tells you the medication slightly improves your vision as long as you keep yourself chronically sleep-deprived. At the end of the commercial, a quieter voice lists the medication's long-term side effects. One of them is that your vision will become much worse if you ever go back to sleeping a normal amount. Would you ever use that medication? Of course not. You cannot go through life tired. Its temporary benefit is not worth its long-term side effects. Now imagine another commercial. This one is for a mail-order weight-loss meal program that slightly reduces your weight as long as you keep yourself chronically food-deprived. At the end of the commercial a quieter voice goes though the program's side effects. The side effects include making you much heavier if you ever go back to eating a normal amount.

Would you ever use that program? Of course not. You cannot go through life hungry. To escape the superstition of starvation, let's dive deeper into the science of its side effects. My favorite experiment showing the side effects of eating less took place at the University of Geneva and involved three groups of rats all eating the same quality of food.

Normal Group: Adult rats eating normally.

Eat Less Group: Adult rats temporarily losing weight by eating less.

Skinny Group: Young rats who naturally weighted about as much as the adult Eat Less group immediately after this group ate less.

If the study were conducted on humans, the Normal Group would be typical thirty-five-year-old women. The Eat Less Group would be thirty-five-year-old women cutting calories until they fit into their high school jeans. And the Skinny Group would be high school girls who fit into size four jeans without trying.

For the first ten days of the study, the Eat Less Group ate 50% less than usual while the Normal Group ate normally. On the tenth day:

The Skinny Group showed up and ate normally.

The Eat Less Group stopped starving themselves and started eating normally.

The Normal Group kept eating normally.

This went on for twenty-five days and the study ended on day thirty-five.

At the end of the thirty-five day study, the Normal Group had eaten normally for thirty-five days. The Eat Less Group had eaten less for ten days and then normally for twenty-five days. And the Skinny Group had eaten normally for twenty-five days.Which group do you think weighed the most and had the highest body fat percentage at the end? The Skinny Group seems like an easy "no" since they are younger and naturally thinner than the other rats. Traditional fat loss theory would say the Eat Less Group is an easy "no" as well since they ate 50% less for ten days. So the Normal Group weighed the most and had the highest body fat percentage at the end of the study, right?Nope.The Eat Less Group weighed the most and had the highest percent body fat. Even though they ate less for ten days, they were significantly heavier than those who ate normally all the way through. Eating less led the rats to gain—not lose—body fat.MacLean at the University of Colorado describes this general metabolic behavior: "[When we eat less] metabolic adjustments occur...[which] contribute to a large potential energy imbalance that, when the forcible control of energy intake is relieved...results in an exceptionally high rate of weight regain."

Super Accumulation of Fat -

Talk about side effects. Eating less was worse than doing nothing.Why?After our metabolism is starved, its number one priority is restoring all the body fat it lost and then protecting us from starving in the future. Guess how it does that? By storing additional body fat. Researchers call this "fat super accumulation." From researcher E.A. Young at the University of Texas: "These and other studies...strongly suggest that fat super accumulation...after energy restriction is a major factor contributing to relapsing obesity, so often observed in humans."The most disturbing aspect of fat super accumulation is that it does not require us to eat a lot. All we have to do is go back to eating a normal amount. The Eat Less Group in the study gained a massive amount of body fat quickly while eating the same amount as the Normal Group and the Skinny Group. The metabolism was trying to make up for the past losses.There is another reason: eating less slowed the metabolism. Put the same quantity and quality of food and exercise into a slowed-down fat metabolism system, and out comes more body fat.

The University of Geneva researchers discovered that the Eat Less Group's metabolisms were burning body fat over 500% less efficiently and had slowed down by 15% by the end of the study. They remarked: "These investigations provide direct evidence for the existence of a specific metabolic component that contributes to an elevated efficiency of energy utilization during refeeding after low food consumption," or once eating less stops.

Starvation does not make us thin. It makes us stocky, sick, and sad. It's bad for health and it's bad for fat loss. Your body just doesn't work that way. Eating less does not cause fat loss.Want more myths shattered from author Jonathan Bailor? Be sure to check out his new book "The Calorie Myth: How To Eat More, Exercise Less, Lose Weight and Live Better". You may also want to tune into my podcast with Jonathan entitled "Can Some Foods Cripple Your Body's Ability To Burn Fat?" – or you can check out the episode where I was a guest on Jonathan's podcast entitled "A Bit Of Biohacking".

Questions, comments or feedback about how eating less does not cause fat loss? Leave your thoughts below!

51) Why Overeating Doesn't Make You Fat (and What Does):

The human body is designed to gain weight and keep it on at all costs. Our survival depends on it. Until we acknowledge that scientific fact, we will never succeed in achieving and maintaining a healthy weight.Doctors and consumers alike believe that overeating and gluttony are the causes of our obesity epidemic. Science tells a different story: it is not completely your fault you are overweight.Powerful genetic forces control our survival behavior. They are at the root of our weight problems. Our bodies weight control systems were designed to produce dozens of molecules that make us eat more and gain weight whenever we have the chance, not to lose it.We have evolved over hundreds of thousands of generations under conditions of food scarcity, not overabundance. Our genes and molecules that control our eating behavior were shaped by those times.

Basically – we are genetically designed to accumulate fat based on the days when we had to forage for food in the wild. Ignoring that fact becomes hazardous to both our health and our waistlines.Furthermore, the food industry and our government's recommendations are fueling this feeding frenzy. We cannot expect to change our instinctual responses to food any more than we can eliminate a feeling of terror when confronted with danger.Think about this: We have hundreds of genes that protect us from starvation, but very few that protect us from overeating.All seems backward, doesn't it? If we remain genetically engineered to gain weight, then it would seem that we are wired incorrectly.Why would we be designed to overeat and grow fat? It all comes down to the oldest and most primitive part of our brain, our limbic, or "lizard," brain. This is the part of your brain that evolved first, and it's like a reptile's brain. It governs your survival behaviors, creating certain chemical responses that you have no conscious control over.While you might think you are in complete control of your mind, the truth is that you have very little control over the unconscious choices you make when you are surrounded by food.

The key to a healthy metabolism is learning what those responses are, how they are triggered, and how you can stop them. You don't want to put yourself in the position of resisting the lure of a bagel. Your drive to eat it will overwhelm any willpower you might have about losing weight. It is a life-or-death experience in your mind, and the bagel will always win.One of the most important principles of weight loss is never to starve yourself. The question is whether or not you are eating enough of the right calories, not whether or not you are eating too many calories. What you need is a baseline for how much you have to eat to keep your body from going into starvation mode.

The Reason Most Diets Fail -

The reason diets backfire almost all the time is because people restrict too much. That is to say, they allow the number of calories they consume to drop below their resting metabolic rate. This is the basic amount of energy or calories needed to run your metabolism for the day. For the average person it is about 10 times your weight in pounds. This is the baseline daily need for your body to simply exist (meaning stay in bed and don't expend any energy). That's not realistic for most of us.If you eat less than that amount (which is what most diets mandate), your body instantly perceives danger and turns on the alarm system that protects you from starvation, slowing your metabolism. As a consequence, your body goes into starvation mode and triggers the signal to eat. So you start eating and eating, and inevitably, you stop the diet — it's the classic rebound weight gain scenario.Just think of what happens when you skip breakfast, work through lunch, and finally return home in the evening: you eat everything in sight. Then you feel stuffed, sick, and guilty and you regret ever entering the kitchen in the first place.

Why would you possibly want to overeat and make yourself sick? Most of us are reasonable people and know that we shouldn't overeat. We have done it before, wished we hadn't, and vowed never to do it again.Nonetheless, time after time, we repeat the same mistakes. Are we weak-willed, morally corrupt, and self-destructive? Do we need years of therapy?The answer is "none of the above." The answer is in our genetic programming. This stuff is just too deep inside us to get away from. We are built to put on weight, and our bodies don't like it very much when we don't give them the calories they need.To make matters worse, when you lose weight, only about half of what is lost is fat; the rest is valuable, metabolically active muscle! Yet when someone regains weight, it is nearly complete fat. Remember, muscle cells burn 70 times more calories than fat cells. Therefore yo-yo dieting makes you lose a big part of your metabolic engine.We all know overweight people who say, "I don't really eat that much, and I still can't lose weight." They aren't lying. When most people go on a diet, they are generally actually making themselves fatter. Each time they diet, they lose muscle.

The diet usually fails, and when it does, the weight that is regained is fat. If you have been through a number of diets that have failed, your body has been through this process a number of times. In short, dieting makes you fat.You want to get away from the diet mentality. What you are undertaking is a way of eating, not a diet.

The Problem with Willpower -

Whatever happened to old-fashioned willpower? Everybody knows that the obesity epidemic is a matter of personal responsibility. People should exercise more self-control. They should avoid overeating and reduce their intake of sugar-sweetened drinks and processed food. There are no good foods or bad foods; it's everything in moderation. Right?This sounds good in theory, except for one thing: New discoveries in science prove that processed, sugar-, fat-, and salt-laden food—food that is made in a plant rather than grown on a plant—is biologically addictive.Remember the old potato chip commercial with the tag line "Bet you can't eat just one"? Bet you can't imagine that kind of commercial for broccoli or apples. No one binges on those foods. Yet it's easy to imagine a mountain of potato chips, a whole bag of cookies, or a pint of ice cream vanishing quickly in an unconscious, reptilian-brain eating frenzy. Broccoli is not addictive, but chips, cookies, ice cream, and soda can become as addictive as any drug.

In the 1980s, First Lady Nancy Reagan championed the "just say no" approach to drug addiction. Unfortunately, that approach hasn't fared too well, and it won't work for our industrial food addiction either. There are specific biological mechanisms that drive addictive behavior.Nobody chooses to be a heroin addict, cokehead, or alcoholic. Nobody chooses to have a food addiction either. These behaviors arise from primitive neurochemical reward centers in the brain that override normal willpower and, in the case of food addictions, overwhelm the ordinary biological signals that control hunger.Why is it so hard for obese people to lose weight despite the social stigma; despite the health consequences such as high blood pressure, diabetes, heart disease, arthritis, and even cancer; and despite their intense desire to lose weight?

Not because they want to be fat. It is because in the vast majority of cases, certain types of food—processed foods made of sugar, fat, and salt combined in ways kept secret by the food industry—are addictive. We are biologically wired to crave these foods and eat as much of them as possible.

52) 10 Strategies to Stop Overeating and Lose Weight:

Fortunately, a number of tips can help you normalize your eating, so that you neither overeat nor under-eat. Thankfully, none of them involve counting calories (or counting anything!). Among the strategies that have helped thousands of my patients lose weight, keep it off, and reduce their risk for diabesity include:Cut out the processed stuff and eat real, whole foods. The single most important thing to lose weight and avoid overeating is to include as many real, whole, unprocessed foods in your diet as possible. Starting right now, make the switch to these foods to lose weight: vegetables, fruits, whole grains, beans, nuts, seeds, olive oil, organic, range, or grass-fed animal products (poultry, lamb, beef, pork, eggs), and wild, smaller fish such as salmon.

Eat breakfast. Skipping breakfast means you're eventually starving, and throughout the day you eat much more food than needed to feel full. To optimize health and weight loss, you need to eat breakfast, to spread out food intake evenly throughout the day, and to not eat for at least two hours before bed. A recent study found that almost 3,000 people who lost an average of 70 pounds and kept it off for six years ate breakfast regularly. Only four percent of people who never ate breakfast kept the weight off.

Eat mindfully. We need to be in a relaxed state for the nervous system of our gut or digestive system to work properly. Eating while we are stressed out makes us fat, both because we don't digest our food properly and because stress hormones slow metabolism and promote fat storage, especially of belly fat. We also tend to overeat when we eat quickly, because it takes the stomach 20 minutes to signal the brain that we are full.Moderate or eliminate alcohol. Taking a holiday from alcohol, besides getting rid of additional sugar calories, will help you tune in to your true appetite and prevent you from overeating.Become aware of trigger foods. For some of us, that one little soda can set us on a downward spiral to overeating and all of the negative health consequences that come with it. It isn't just the processed, sugary foods and drinks that become triggers. But even healthy foods, if you have a tendency to binge on them, can quickly become unhealthy. A handful of almonds are perfectly healthy, but if you eat half the jar, they quickly become unhealthy.

Keep a Journal. Journaling is an excellent way to get in touch with your inner motivations, to break the cycle of mindless eating and activity, to be honest and accountable and present to yourself. We often overeat because something is eating away at us. We stuff ourselves with food in order to stuff our feelings away. We use food to block feelings, but you can use words to block food. You can write in order to better metabolize your feelings so they don't end up driving unconscious choices or overeating. A diet of words and self-exploration often results in weight loss. You metabolize your life and calories better.Get sufficient sleep. Get eight hours of quality, uninterrupted sleep every night. You'll find that you're less prone to cravings and you will normalize fat-regulating hormones. One study found even a partial night's sleep deprivation contributes to insulin resistance, paving the way for obesity and type 2 diabetes.Control stress levels. Most of us fail to notice the effects of the chronic stresses we live with every day: demanding jobs, marital tension, lack of sleep, too much to do and too little time to do it. I am sure the list goes on for many. Chronic stress makes us overeat, not to mention overeating the wrong kinds of food, which ultimately leads to weight gain. Learn to actively relax with meditation, yoga, deep breathing, or any other technique that helps you reduce stress.

Exercise the right way. You can't over-exercise your way out of a bad diet, but the right exercise can help you lose weight, maintain weight loss, and control your appetite so you don't overeat. Ideally you should do a minimum of 30 minutes of walking every day. Get a pedometer to track your steps. Wear it every day and set a goal of 10,000 steps a day. More vigorous and sustained exercise is often needed to reverse severe obesity and diabesity. Run, bike, dance, play games, jump on a trampoline, or do whatever is fun for you. Read this blog for a comprehensive, easy-to-implement exercise plan.

Supplement smartly. Obesity and diabetes are often paradoxically states of malnutrition. It has been said that diabetes is starvation in the midst of plenty. The sugar can't get into the cells. Your metabolism is sluggish, and the cells don't communicate as a finely tuned team. Nutrients are an essential part of getting back in balance and correcting the core problem— insulin resistance.

If you would like to cut-out the processed food, stop mindless eating and learn how to cook delicious, whole-food recipes, then download the sneak preview of my newest book, releasing on March 10th, The 10-Day Detox Diet Cookbook. In addition to the recipes you will also learn about the secret added ingredient that keeps you hooked on junk food! Click here to get this sneak preview now.

53) 10 weight loss secrets from around the world :

What are the favourite ways to get and stay slim across the globe? We look at some of the most popular and get lowdown from a dietician to see if they're worth a try.Sometimes we need to look further afield than our fridge to find the answers to our weight loss dreams, which is why we scanned the globe to find out what dieters in other countries do to slim down.To save everyone time and money – (plus nobody wants to be downing turmeric shots for no good reason (see number 7) – we spoke to Kiri Elliott, dietitian and media spokesperson for the British Dietetic Association, to suss out whether these tactics are worth trying for yourself.

Here Are 10 weight loss secrets from around the world

a) Pu'er tea in China-

You might be wondering what pu'er tea is and ironically, the clue is in the name. It's a fermented tea that promotes bowel movement and weight loss. In China, they tend to drink it after a large meal to aid digestion. And they are quite specific about the timing – around one hour after you've finished eating. Kiri says: 'In the case of Pu-er tea, the contents and size of the meal eaten are likely to have a much greater effect on weight loss goals than the tea drunk after it! There is limited scientific evidence that any teas actually work, and people need to be cautious as well as high levels of caffeine, some teas contain herbs that in too high doses have side effects such as dehydration, electrolyte imbalance and can damage the gut.'You might be wondering what pu'er tea is and ironically, the clue is in the name. It's a fermented tea that promotes bowel movement and weight loss. In China, they tend to drink it after a large meal to aid digestion. And they are quite specific about the timing – around one hour after you've finished eating.

Kiri says: 'In the case of Pu-er tea, the contents and size of the meal eaten are likely to have a much greater effect on weight loss goals than the tea drunk after it! There is limited scientific evidence that any teas actually work, and people need to be cautious as well as high levels of caffeine, some teas contain herbs that in too high doses have side effects such as dehydration, electrolyte imbalance and can damage the gut.'

b) Rice and beans in Brazil-

Brazilians may manage to stay slim due to indulging in a traditional dish of rice and beans. 'They eat it with just about meal,' Sergio Charlab, editor of Reader's Digest Brazil, explains. And a recent study, published in the Obesity Research journal, supports this. Scientists found that a diet consisting primarily of rice and beans lowers the risk of becoming overweight by about 14% when compared with the food we typically eat here. That's because it's lower in fat and higher in fibre.Kiri says: 'Rice and beans can be a great part of a balanced meal, as they are naturally low in fat and high in fibre, especially if wholegrain rice is used rather than the traditional white rice which is staple in Brazil. However the key really is in the preparation.'The other thing is that size of portion will have a large effect on weight loss goals and that for a healthy balanced diet the rice and beans should be part of the meal (they can contributing the main source of carbs and protein of that meal) and not an additional accompaniment.'Brazilians may manage to stay slim due to indulging in a traditional dish of rice and beans. 'They eat it with just about meal,' Sergio Charlab, editor of Reader's Digest Brazil, explains. And a recent study, published in the Obesity Research journal, supports this. Scientists found that a diet consisting primarily of rice and beans lowers the risk of becoming overweight by about 14% when compared with the food we typically eat here. That's because it's lower in fat and higher in fibre.

Kiri says: 'Rice and beans can be a great part of a balanced meal, as they are naturally low in fat and high in fibre, especially if wholegrain rice is used rather than the traditional white rice which is staple in Brazil. However the key really is in the preparation.

'The other thing is that size of portion will have a large effect on weight loss goals and that for a healthy balanced diet the rice and beans should be part of the meal (they can contributing the main source of carbs and protein of that meal) and not an additional accompaniment.'

c) Yoga in India-

It may not be the high-intensity workout we are told will burn tons of calories but it research shows it does still facilitate weight loss. In a study carried out at North Central University in America, scientists found that those who regularly practiced yoga had a lower body mass index than those who engaged in other forms of exercise. Yoga is muscle building, boosts your metabolism and encourages you to tune into your body. Yogis often comment on how many of the poses aid digestion and also help them become more mindful of when they are full. Kiri says: 'To lose weight the body needs to use up more calories than it takes in and one way to shift the balance is via more movement and exercise. The best results for long-term weight loss happen when activity levels are increased and that this increase becomes part of lifestyle for the long term.'

It may not be the high-intensity workout we are told will burn tons of calories but it research shows it does still facilitate weight loss. In a study carried out at North Central University in America, scientists found that those who regularly practiced yoga had a lower body mass index than those who engaged in other forms of exercise. Yoga is muscle building, boosts your metabolism and encourages you to tune into your body. Yogis often comment on how many of the poses aid digestion and also help them become more mindful of when they are full.

Kiri says: 'To lose weight the body needs to use up more calories than it takes in and one way to shift the balance is via more movement and exercise. The best results for long-term weight loss happen when activity levels are increased and that this increase becomes part of lifestyle for the long term.'

d) Herring in Norway-

The Dutch love herring – they eat around 85 million of them per year. They're particularly enjoyed lightly pickled, served as snacks or in bread. So, why could herring be good for weight loss? For starters it's an oily fish, which helps reduce stress due to its omega-3 fatty acids. Cortisol, the stress hormone, is known to increase the amount of visceral fat we gain around our tums. As well as this, it's just simple maths. Herring is low in calories – so swapping your usual sandwich filling for this fishy alternative is going to have an impact on your weight loss. Kiri says: 'Oily fish are known for their omega-3 content and the benefits of these are related to heart health and many, such as herring, include vitamin A, D and protein. However, there is no substantial evidence to suggest that oily fish keeps our waistlines slim. We recommend that two portions of fish (140g) should be eaten each week and one of these should be oily.'

The Dutch love herring – they eat around 85 million of them per year. They're particularly enjoyed lightly pickled, served as snacks or in bread. So, why could herring be good for weight loss? For starters it's an oily fish, which helps reduce stress due to its omega-3 fatty acids. Cortisol, the stress hormone, is known to increase the amount of visceral fat we gain around our tums. As well as this, it's just simple maths. Herring is low in calories – so swapping your usual sandwich filling for this fishy alternative is going to have an impact on your weight loss.

Kiri says: 'Oily fish are known for their omega-3 content and the benefits of these are related to heart health and many, such as herring, include vitamin A, D and protein. However, there is no substantial evidence to suggest that oily fish keeps our waistlines slim. We recommend that two portions of fish (140g) should be eaten each week and one of these should be oily.'

e) Rooibos tea in South Africa-

Swapping your afternoon cuppa for a rooibos tea (also known as redbush tea) could be a good way to cut calories from your day and give you the sugary hit you need. South African's enjoy a cup of the naturally sweet drink which helps reduce cravings and is a good afternoon go-to instead of a handful of biscuits. Kiri says: 'Again, back to the teatoxing! The way Rooibos could work here is more about the added ingredients to the great British cuppa! A traditional cup of tea with milk and sugar has around 40 calories per cup. If this is swapped to Rooibos taken without milk and sugar then that's a saving of 40 calories per cup. Over the course of a day, 4-5 cups means160-200kcal/day.'

Swapping your afternoon cuppa for a rooibos tea (also known as redbush tea) could be a good way to cut calories from your day and give you the sugary hit you need. South African's enjoy a cup of the naturally sweet drink which helps reduce cravings and is a good afternoon go-to instead of a handful of biscuits.

Kiri says: 'Again, back to the teatoxing! The way Rooibos could work here is more about the added ingredients to the great British cuppa! A traditional cup of tea with milk and sugar has around 40 calories per cup. If this is swapped to Rooibos taken without milk and sugar then that's a saving of 40 calories per cup. Over the course of a day, 4-5 cups means160-200kcal/day.'

f) Power nap in Japan-

This one sounds too good to be true and might have you packing your belongings to move across the world. Many Japanese people allow time for naps during the day, just a short 20 minutes or so, but it could be the difference between a healthy meal or an evening carb-loading binge. We know that we crave more sugary, high-fat foods when we are sleep deprived and this leads to weight gain. This is because the hormone leptin, which informs the brain when you are full is in low supply in a sleep-deprived body. At the same time levels of ghrelin, the hormone which triggers hunger, rise. 'Many people think they're hungry when they're actually sleepy,' James Maas, sleep researcher at Cornell University, explains. 'Instead of a snack, they need some shut-eye.'So if anyone catches you snoozing, just tell them: 'I wasn't napping, I was dieting'. Kiri says: 'How well we sleep has a huge impact on our overall wellbeing and yes not getting enough sleep plays havoc with our hormones which can make it difficult to understand our hunger and satiety cues. 'Rather than grabbing powernaps here and there, having a regular sleeping pattern is important. Going to bed earlier and having a longer sleep (most people need 6-9 hours per night) is likely to be much better than having a powernap as the body has a chance recuperate properly from the day's activities.'

This one sounds too good to be true and might have you packing your belongings to move across the world. Many Japanese people allow time for naps during the day, just a short 20 minutes or so, but it could be the difference between a healthy meal or an evening carb-loading binge. We know that we crave more sugary, high-fat foods when we are sleep deprived and this leads to weight gain. This is because the hormone leptin, which informs the brain when you are full is in low supply in a sleep-deprived body. At the same time levels of ghrelin, the hormone which triggers hunger, rise. 'Many people think they're hungry when they're actually sleepy,' James Maas, sleep researcher at Cornell University, explains. 'Instead of a snack, they need some shut-eye.'So if anyone catches you snoozing, just tell them: 'I wasn't napping, I was dieting'.

Kiri says: 'How well we sleep has a huge impact on our overall wellbeing and yes not getting enough sleep plays havoc with our hormones which can make it difficult to understand our hunger and satiety cues. 'Rather than grabbing powernaps here and there, having a regular sleeping pattern is important. Going to bed earlier and having a longer sleep (most people need 6-9 hours per night) is likely to be much better than having a powernap as the body has a chance recuperate properly from the day's activities.'

g) Turmeric in Malaysia-

We might add this spice to our curries over here but in Malaysia it is a much more staple part of diet. As well as having anti-inflammatory properties, turmeric also contains something called curcumin, which could be a powerful fat burner. A recent study by researchers at Tufts University in Boston found that mice given small amounts of curcumin alongside a high-fat diet gained less weight then rodents who went without the extra substance. The team believes that this could be proof the ingredient suppresses the growth of fat tissue and increases fat burning. Add it to your cooking or mix with milk to make a turmeric latte. Kiri says: 'Scientists in laboratories are researching the effects of curcumin but as far as evidence in human populations there is a lack of evidence to prove any potential fat burning properties could work safely. Ultimately turmeric is not a miracle spice and people need to be cautious of using high dose supplements until more is known.'

We might add this spice to our curries over here but in Malaysia it is a much more staple part of diet. As well as having anti-inflammatory properties, turmeric also contains something called curcumin, which could be a powerful fat burner. A recent study by researchers at Tufts University in Boston found that mice given small amounts of curcumin alongside a high-fat diet gained less weight then rodents who went without the extra substance. The team believes that this could be proof the ingredient suppresses the growth of fat tissue and increases fat burning.

Add it to your cooking or mix with milk to make a turmeric latte.

Kiri says: 'Scientists in laboratories are researching the effects of curcumin but as far as evidence in human populations there is a lack of evidence to prove any potential fat burning properties could work safely. Ultimately turmeric is not a miracle spice and people need to be cautious of using high dose supplements until more is known.

h) More talking in France-

This is possibly the easiest weight-loss technique we have ever come across: talk more. We couldn't have dreamt up a better diet tip ourselves! The French love a drawn-out dinner, in fact 92% of the countries families dine together nightly. 'For the French, eating is the event of the day,' says Fred Pescatore, MD, president of the International & American Associations of Clinical Nutritionists. 'For us, it's something we do before heading out to do something else.'Kiri says: 'Pausing between bites, chewing food well and eating slowly definitely gives us a better chance of recognising our satiety cues before we over indulge. Whilst some people find distraction from the food like eating with family helps them to eat more slowly, many find that eating with others is a distraction and are more likely get engrossed in conversation and could miss the satiety signals.'This is possibly the easiest weight-loss technique we have ever come across: talk more. We couldn't have dreamt up a better diet tip ourselves!

The French love a drawn-out dinner, in fact 92% of the countries families dine together nightly.

'For the French, eating is the event of the day,' says Fred Pescatore, MD, president of the International & American Associations of Clinical Nutritionists. 'For us, it's something we do before heading out to do something else.'Kiri says: 'Pausing between bites, chewing food well and eating slowly definitely gives us a better chance of recognising our satiety cues before we over indulge. Whilst some people find distraction from the food like eating with family helps them to eat more slowly, many find that eating with others is a distraction and are more likely get engrossed in conversation and could miss the satiety signals.'

i) Pickles in Hungary-

If you're a fan of all things pickled then chances are you'll love Hungary. They are a nation of vinegar lovers it seems and happily crunch on copious amounts of pickled peppers, cabbage and tomatoes. It has been widely reported that drinking apple cider vinegar can aid weight loss but is it worth stocking up on jars of the stuff? Kiri says: 'A study carried out on Japanese participants in 2009 found that people who weighed around 11.5 stone lost 2-4lb by drinking a small amount of diluted cider vinegar each day. It took these participants 12 weeks to lose that much weight and the results were not sustained after the three months mark. 'As a dietitian I would not consider this much weigh loss clinically significant for health and know of other ways to achieve better sustainable weight loss for health and wellbeing.'

But what about tucking into some nice pickled carrot? 'There is no evidence to suggest that pickles assist with weight loss. However switching a creamy coleslaws or potato salad to a couple of pickled onions or gherkins could save a few calories!'If you're a fan of all things pickled then chances are you'll love Hungary. They are a nation of vinegar lovers it seems and happily crunch on copious amounts of pickled peppers, cabbage and tomatoes. It has been widely reported that drinking apple cider vinegar can aid weight loss but is it worth stocking up on jars of the stuff?

Kiri says: 'A study carried out on Japanese participants in 2009 found that people who weighed around 11.5 stone lost 2-4lb by drinking a small amount of diluted cider vinegar each day. It took these participants 12 weeks to lose that much weight and the results were not sustained after the three months mark. 'As a dietitian I would not consider this much weigh loss clinically significant for health and know of other ways to achieve better sustainable weight loss for health and wellbeing.'

But what about tucking into some nice pickled carrot? 'There is no evidence to suggest that pickles assist with weight loss. However switching a creamy coleslaws or potato salad to a couple of pickled onions or gherkins could save a few calories!'

j) Fasting in Indonesia-

Those familiar with the 5:2 diet may already know about the benefits of intermittent fasting but in Indonesia they called it Mutih. During Mutih, Indonesians eat only white rice and drink only water. Though it is not intended for weight loss fasting, or cutting your calories in half, for a day or two is a great way to make you more mindful of how much you are eating. It gives your digestive system a chance to clear out and improve its efficiency – leading to weight loss. Kiri says: 'Unless properly managed a fasting diet is likely to lead to a lack of concentration, tiredness and low mood. Depending on your age, health and lifestyle, fasting can also be dangerous. Tiredness and low mood can also have a negative effect on food choices once fasting has finished.'If you want to go down the fasting route for weight loss, it is important to choose an evidence-based plan and consult a medical professional to ensure that this is done in a healthy and safe way.'

Those familiar with the 5:2 diet may already know about the benefits of intermittent fasting but in Indonesia they called it Mutih. During Mutih, Indonesians eat only white rice and drink only water. Though it is not intended for weight loss fasting, or cutting your calories in half, for a day or two is a great way to make you more mindful of how much you are eating. It gives your digestive system a chance to clear out and improve its efficiency – leading to weight loss. Kiri says: 'Unless properly managed a fasting diet is likely to lead to a lack of concentration, tiredness and low mood. Depending on your age, health and lifestyle, fasting can also be dangerous. Tiredness and low mood can also have a negative effect on food choices once fasting has finished.

'If you want to go down the fasting route for weight loss, it is important to choose an evidence-based plan and consult a medical professional to ensure that this is done in a healthy and safe way.'

53) 9 places to take a weight-loss vacation:

When it comes to serious weight loss, many people are swapping their regular holiday for a weight loss vacation.By cutting off distractions to everyday life and work, these trips offer individualized fitness and diet plans intended to last well beyond a week or two.Today's best weight loss vacations offer fitness adventure, spa detoxing, or medical programs to help people reach their weight loss goals through good food, engaged activities and proven medical advice.

Here Are 9 places to take a weight-loss vacation

a) The Ranch, Live Oak Malibu, United States-

The Ranch at Live Oak Malibu gives a one-week full immersion bootcamp in the heart of nature. The 120-acre Ranch is a fitness retreat set three miles above the Pacific Ocean in the Santa Monica Mountains.The program is designed to help participants gain physical endurance, lose weight, detoxify, and learn how to keep the weight off once they get back on the grid.

Some 2,000 participants on the program have lost an average of 8.82 lbs. a week and women lose an average of 5.09 lbs. a week.The program focuses on sustainable exercise such as daily hikes, yoga, and core work with weights. The intense day is jam-packed from 5.30 a.m. to 7 p.m., with 8-10 hours of exercise in-between, but there's always time for a daily nap and massage.

Austin Ligon, a former CEO, went to the Ranch three times this past year, maintaining a loss of 15 pounds of body fat. "It makes weight loss easy," he says, "because you don't have to work out your own program and stick to it. You just join the group, do the week, and see how it comes out."The menu of organic vegetarian cuisine is limited to 1,400 calories a day using ingredients picked daily from the Ranch's own gardens. Example meals include Zucchini Fettuccini with Cauliflower Bolognese, Sunflower Seed Risotto and Hearts of Palm

Crab Cakes

The seven-day Ranch program, which includes full room and board, daily activities and massages, is held weekly (Sun-Sat) and costs $6,200; +1 310 457 8700; theranchmalibu.com

b) Lefay Resort & Spa, Lake Garda, Italy-

Beautiful setting, inside and outside.courtesy lefay resort and spa Set at the top of Lake Garda, Italy's largest and most scenic lake, Lefay Resort & Spa is an eco resort covering 3,000 square meters and featuring indoor and outdoor heated salt-water pools, a 10% indoor salt lake, five types of saunas and a crushed ice fountain.At the heart of Lefay Spa is Dr. Maurizio Corradin, a Western-trained, Eastern-practicing doctor. His philosophy is simple: "You must enjoy life," and he believes any diet that puts heavy restrictions on a person is bound to fail.

Rather than focus on food restrictions, they focus on what guests can eat, using only ingredients the guest chooses. His treatment program follows Chinese Medicine in order to to restore optimal flows of Qi (energy) in order to set the body and mind on the right path toward achieving its optimal weight.Corradin designed a series of Tui Na massages in order to solve specific problems such as draining excess fluid, improving sleep or curing sugar cravings. His foot reflexology stimulates meridians or energetic lines to detox and regulate the body.Corradin uses aromatic hydrotherapy to treat stress and tension. He may also prescribe acupuncture, and moxibustion heat treatments, as well as phytotheraphy, or medicinal teas.Daily exercise classes are encouraged, including the Meridian stretches, Tai Qi and Qi-Gong for stress relief, as well as water gym classes and Pilates to increase energy.

The Slimming and Weight Loss Program is available exclusively through Wellbeing Escapes at Lefay Spa and costs from £1,815 ($2,982)/per person for a min five night's stay inclusive of doctor consultation, all massage and energy treatments, accommodation,

full board and activities; +44 207 644 6111;
www.wellbeingescapes.com

c) Fitness Travel, Senegal-

Fitness Travel Company designs itineraries for guests to explore a new country and get in top physical shape at the same time.Upcoming trips include a Senegal adventure where guests will embark on an action-packed week full of beach runs, an 18-mile cycle to a lion cub game reserve, kayaking to a private beach and learning African dance to the sound of local drums.To maximize weight loss, guests will eat a high-protein/low-carb Paleolithic-inspired diet, starting the day with a fresh juice and continuing with alkalizing raw fruit and vegetables and fresh seafood. The trip fee includes an in-depth personal training course in the guest's home country, three weeks in advance in order to prepare for the trip, and one week on return.

Spandana Gopal, a business owner in London, recently went on the Senegal trip and lost 5.5 lbs. with the pre-month training, and her husband lost 9 lbs. "The experience was fantastic," she says. "I think the fact that I can see a different country and stay fit at the same time made me love the trip."A Thailand trip Involves deep jungle running in Chiang Mai, Muay Thai training, mountain biking through remote villages and Thai cooking lessons.A Masai Wild Warrior fitness trip in Nairobi lets guests train like warriors through tree climbing, game walks, spear throwing, hill sprints and bush crawling. And a ladies-only slimming retreat in Bodrum lets women learn flyboarding, wind surfing and water skiing in Turkey's most beautiful, blue peninsula.

A seven-day all-inclusive package including accommodation, all activities, meals, transfers in Senegal, tours and sightseeing is £2,450 ($4.034) based on two people sharing; Single supplement £350; +44 800 001 6409; www.fitnesstravelcompany.com

d) Ti Sana, Lombardy, Italy-

Ti Sana is a small 22-suite, family-owned retreat in Lecco a 50-kilometer drive north of Milan. The resort is a former 18th century home with stone country walls and a state-of-the-art spa.Upon arrival, guests of the Healtheatarian, Active Life Program, undergo a series of tests to measure the body's current level of health and stress. The spa's staff then develops an individualized exercise and nutrition plan in order to make guests aware of how to optimize energy.Ti Sana's weight loss program is somewhat extreme for diet novices, but guarantees fat loss over muscle and water weight loss as well as reducing other issues such as poor digestion.

Participants can choose between a juice cleanse or a raw food diet, consisting of small portions of vegetable-heavy foods.Caffeine, flour, sugar and other staples are not allowed on the program. Ti Sana claims that after one week, cravings for sugar and processed foods disappear, and energy levels go through the roof.Daily fitness includes a walk around the nearby lake as well as several exercise classes, from trampoline rebounding to muscle hypertrophy.To counteract the intense programming guests have access to a beautiful underground spa that combines a wide range of healing hydrotherapy from saline pools to rainforest and mint showers with a great selection of hot saunas including infrared and steam rooms.Guests leave with a personalized diet as well as the Ti Sana "Manual for an Active Life," which provides a step-by-step approach to how to maintain the results gained from the detox, living the Mediterrean diet, advice on natural beauty routines and a guide to physical activity.

The Healtheatarian Program includes suite accommodation, beauty and medical spa treatments, full board physical activities and lectures, starting from €3,710 ($5,045) for a 10-night stay; +39 9920979; www.1711.it

e) Canyon Ranch, Tucson, United States-

Walk your way to health.courtesy the ranch.A former cattle ranch located on 150 acres in the Sonoran Desert, Tucson's Canyon Ranch is a mainstay in health and wellness and celebrates its 35th anniversary this year."It's a program for people tired of fad diets who are ready to embrace a lifestyle approach. We moved away from the bootcamp fat farm approach of weigh loss vacations to more of a lifestyle management course," says Jim Eastburn, life enhancement director at Canyon Ranch.

What sets Canyon Ranch apart is its large medical faculty. It employs over 60 wellness professionals, including integrative medicine physicians, clinical grade nutritionists, exercise physiologists, spirituality practitioners and licensed behavioral therapists.Guests undergo a series of medical assessments. Their program director then designs an individualized nutrition and fitness course. Therapists work with guests to address lifestyle variables and emotional issues that may be affecting their results, aiming to teach them how to reprioritize behaviors to put their health first.There are daily lectures that address topics like one's relationship with food, brain fitness, healthy eating on the go and maximizing your metabolism.

Susan Earl, a retired special education director, says of the experience, "I not only lost 42 pounds, but I reversed my recent diagnosis of Diabetes as well as lowered all of my previously high cholesterol and triglyceride numbers into the healthy range. I honestly believe I could not have done this if I had not participated in their program."

A seven-day single-stay all-inclusive package starts at $8,650; +1 520 749 9000; www.canyonranch.com

f) Talise Spa, Madinat Jumeriah, Dubai, U.A.E. -

Talise Spa at Madinat Jumeriah has a reputation for not only being one of the best spas in the world, but for having the most integrated medical weight loss solution offered in the Middle East.Guests who arrive at the spa meet with doctors to determine first why they're carrying excess pounds. An initial consultation includes a full body scan as well as in-depth blood tests that may lead to further testing.If the extra weight comes from a careless diet and bad eating habits, doctors will do a blood analysis to check cholesterol levels and triglycerides. If metabolism is low, guests will undergo a series of food intolerance tests.

Common diagnoses are hormonal imbalances, metobolical dysfunctions, sugar imbalances, lack of exercise and food cravings from emotional imbalance.A typical program may begin with a liver and intensive detox, and then followed up with a variety of treatments such as sessions in the infrared sauna, relaxing yoga and tai chi or strength-building kung fu classes, and a course of homeopathic medications, supplements and vitamins.The resort wellness chef designs a meal plan for the guest's length of stay, which depending on the guest's diagnosis, may be a low GI diet, a high protein diet or a diuretic diet.Internal medicine specialist Dr. Elisabeth Makk at Talise Spa says, "A holistic weight loss program is designed for those that are ready to make a change, not just to their diet, but also in their lifestyle. It's about understanding your strengths and limitations, and concentrating on prevention, focus and renewal."

An initial consultation costs AED 1700 ($462), and the individualized plan is developed from there; a one-week stay at Madinet Jumeirah starts at AED 16,380 ($4,600); +971 4 366 6818; www.jumeirah.com

g) Thermia Palace, Slovakia-

The Art Nouveau Thermia Palace in Piešťany, Slovakia, has for over 100 years welcomed anyone from kings, sheiks and czars, all wanting to experience the sulfur-rich thermal mineral waters and healing mud sources on the spa island.The 20-strong medical staff in Piešťany focus on wellness and weight loss, aiming to become once again Europe's top medical spa.Its one-week slimming spa stay program includes a doctor consultation and health examinations including metabolic functioning, nutrition planning, fitness training and a wide assortment of doctor-prescribed therapies (up to 30 a week), such as hydromassages and medical massages to increase blood circulation.

Guests can have a sulfur mud bath under the stained-glass windows to target specific problem areas. The slimming program focuses not only on diet and fitness, but also on preventing damage to joints and to the body. Natural springs have been proven to aid in diseases such as rheumatism, and also give incredible energy and strength to anyone coming to kickoff a fitness lifestyle."With the pharmaceutical industry, it's not well-known if the treatments will last, or what kind of long-term damage is being done," says CEO Klaus Pilz, who says their programs are so effective that over 50% of repeat guests visit at least once a year. "As a medical spa, the only side effects of our treatments are sore muscles after a massage."

Weight Loss at Thermia Palace is a unique program designed by Wellbeing Escapes and costs from £902 ($1,482)/per person for a seven-night stay inclusive of all spa treatments, fitness classes, luxury accommodation and meals; +44 207 644 6111; www.wellbeingescapes.com

South Korea's most outrageous sauna: Spa Land Centum City

h) Absolute Sanctuary, Koh Samui, Thailand-

The takeaway from this Thai establishment? Suppleness.courtesy absolute santuaryAbsolute Sanctuary is a boutique resort overlooking the Cheong Mon Peninsula."Familiarity breeds contempt," says Claire Bostock, executive director of Absolute Sanctuary. "Take that away and things get easier. Plus, in an island such as Koh Samui, known as the island of healing, just the atmosphere itself makes one motivated to keep to their goals."Guests can choose between a seven, 10, or 14-day program, and lose an average of 6.5-22 lbs., according to Bostock. The most she saw was a CEO of a multinational firm who lost 20 lbs. in 10 days, down from 375 lbs., by following the resort's diet menu and program activities.

Light meals are chosen with organic handpicked local produce, cold-pressed oils and whole-food seasonings and superfoods like flaxseeds, spirulina and coconut oil. A sample menu could be an apple and guava omega fruit salad for breakfast, cashew brown rice stir-fry for lunch, and raw Pad Thai for dinner.Absolute Sanctuary's two-fold fitness approach offers tailored physical exercises from Pilates to fit ball to endurance and resistance training. It combines exercise with cleansing mental therapies such as hypnotherapy and Reiki designed to break down any emotional barriers to weight loss.

The standard one-week course includes multiple spa sessions, full room and board and fitness classes, from THB 96,900 ($2,937); +66 77 601 205; www.absolutesanctuary.com

i) Rancho La Puerta, Mexico-

Just across the border in Tecate, Mexico, at the juncture of the Laguna and Sierra Juarez mountain ranges, is Rancho La Puerta, a 3,000-acre resort full of gardens, mountains and meadows.A week at the ranch teaches sustainable nutritional eating and muscle building. "If guests exercise in moderation during their stay and eat the servings we provide, they can expect to lost 2-5 lbs. in the week," says Yvonne Nienstadt, director of nutrition at Rancho La Puerta.Dubbing their weight-loss diet the "Mexo-Mediterrenean Diet," the Ranch's menu is largely based on plants and whole foods, banning all processed food. Calories are reduced moderately, not radically in order to lose fat and not muscle.

Nienstadt recalls one guest, Suzanne, who lost 24 pounds over three weeks by eating huge salads, drinking fresh green juices and cutting out dairy, gluten and sugar."People then feel better, and feel like eating right rather than self medicating with 'comfort foods' and they feel like getting up off the couch and exercising," says Nienstadt."Within four days Suzanne told me her knees were no longer hurting and she could exercise more freely and by the end of three weeks, she stated that not only did she feel lighter physically, but mentally she felt 'high.'"Rancho La Puerto has over 40 daily activities, from high intensity interval training, bird walk, cardio drumming, hula hooping, African dance, Feldenkrais, tennis clinic, and meditation workshops.

A seven-night stay, single occupancy, begin at $3,650, which covers accommodations, meals, fitness classes and presentations; +1 858 764 5500; www.rancholapuerta.com

54) You Asked: What's the Best Way to Lose 5 Pounds Fast?

You've heard (over and over again) that gradual weight loss is sustainable weight loss. And you're totally going to incorporate all of those healthy lifestyle changes that will help you shed your extra pounds and keep them off for good.But you'll start all that next month. This month, you've got your friend's wedding and a beach weekend to worry about. So what's the best way to lose five pounds fast?Start by ditching salt, says Dana Hunnes, a senior clinical dietitian at UCLA Medical Center. "The average American eats about 4,000 mg of sodium a day, and that can cause you to retain a lot of water weight," she explains. "Just cutting your sodium way down can help you lose three, four, five pounds very quickly."

To do that, you'll want to avoid all packaged products—including cured or deli meats—all of which tend to be loaded with salt. Hunnes says anything under 1,500 mg a day is "really good," but if you can go lower sticking with fresh foods, even better.Also on the chopping block: processed carbohydrates. Think breads, pastas, fruit juices and pretty much all snack or dessert foods. "Carbs are hydrophilic molecules, meaning they love water," Hunnes says. "They make it more difficult for your body to release water from your kidneys through metabolism."By ditching both processed carbs and cutting way back on sodium, you'll lose weight, and it will be the kind around your midsection that people will really be able to notice. "With water weight, you can be bloated and not realize it," Hunnes says. "I have people do this and say, 'I can see my abs for the first time!'"Two important warnings here: If you're not completely healthy, talk to your doctor before making any changes to your diet, Hunnes says.

Also, if you're exercising a lot while you're trying to lose weight—especially if you sweat a ton when you work out—you need to be careful about slashing salt too severely. Sodium is one of the electrolytes your body loses when you sweat. If you're adding an intense exercise program to your low-salt diet in order to lose weight, you could be at risk for hyponatremia, a potentially life-threatening condition linked with heavy sweating, heavy water intake and too-little sodium consumption.

55) 9 Science-Backed Weight Loss Tips:

Losing weight is tough, both mentally and physically. New science shows that when the body starts to lose substantial amounts of weight, it fights viciously to gain it back. But despite the biological roadblocks, plenty of people are successful at losing weight and keeping it off over the long term.But how? As part of its recent exploration of the new science of weight loss, TIME asked 9 weight loss and obesity experts their best advice for people who are trying to lose weight.

Here are their top tips for what works when it comes to slimming down

a) Don't focus on calories-

"The 'calorie in, calorie out' approach fails, because it disregards how food affects our hormones and metabolism. Pay attention to food quality."

—Dr. David S. Ludwig, professor of nutrition at Harvard Medical School

b) Keep it basic-

"The simple message is to eat a healthful diet and to engage in more moderate-to-vigorous physical activity. The challenge is how to actually accomplish that in an environment that seems to push us constantly in the wrong direction."

—Dr. Stephen R. Daniels, pediatrician-in-chief at Children's Hospital Colorado

c)Adjust your goal weight-

"Aim to achieve and improve health and reach a psychologically 'happy weight,' not an unrealistic 'ideal' weight that may be impossible to reach for most."

—Dr. Jaideep Behari, associate professor of medicine at the University of Pittsburgh School of Medicine

d) Commit to change-

"People need to have the mindset of someone who is ready and willing to make some permanent changes in the way they live. A number of treatments can create short-term weight loss without a great deal of effort from the person, but they don't allow for long-term weight loss."

—Dr. Michael Jensen, obesity researcher at the Mayo Clinic

e) Eat delicious food-

"You need a program that satisfies hunger and has good food so it doesn't feel like a diet. Hunger erodes willpower, and that's the reason most diets fail."

—Susan B. Roberts, professor of nutrition at Tufts University and founder of iDiet

f) Recruit support-

"Make small changes that stick, make changes as a family and keep it positive."

—Dr. Stephen Pont, medical director of the childhood obesity center at Dell Children's Medical Center

g) Get educated-

"The culprit is not bad choices by individuals. It is the toxic food environment in which calories are ubiquitous. Until the food environment changes, everyone must become aware of the calories they consume, especially those from beverages, sweets, and other calorie-dense foods."

—Dr. Lawrence J. Appel, director of the Welch Center for Prevention, Epidemiology, and Clinical Research at Johns Hopkins University

h) Make friends with moderation-

"A person can eat almost anything they want, but the portion size has to be appropriate. For example, eat dinner on a salad plate rather than a dinner plate to cut the portion size in half."

—Melinda L. Irwin, professor of epidemiology at Yale School of Public

Health

i) Cut out soda-

"Avoid all sugary drinks, as they provide 'empty calories' that don't fill you up. The sugar may uniquely act on the liver to produce belly fat."

—Dr. Dean Schillinger, chief of the University of California, San Francisco Division of General Internal Medicine.